ANATOMY OF A DOG PAW

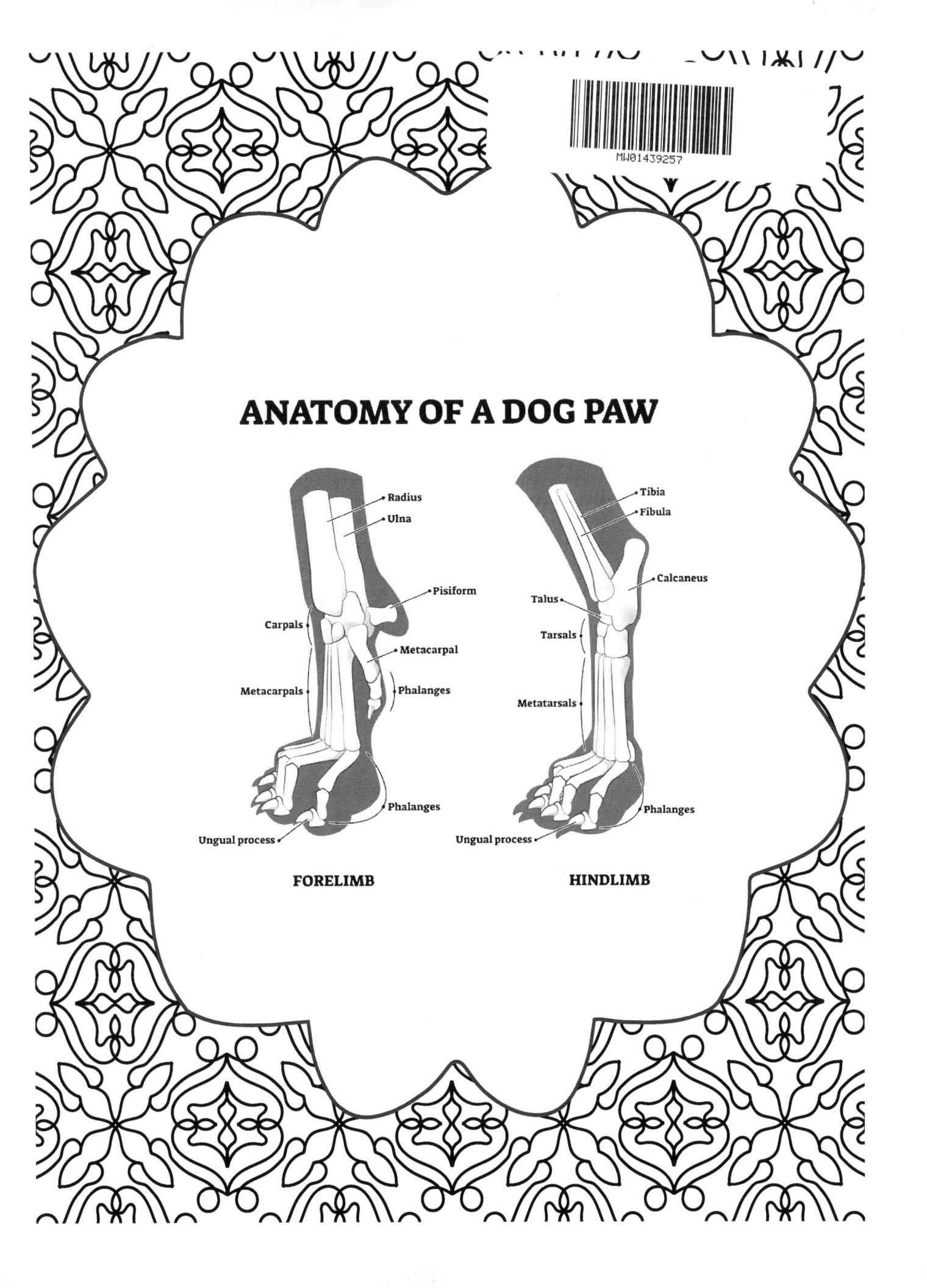

FORELIMB

- Radius
- Ulna
- Pisiform
- Carpals
- Metacarpal
- Metacarpals
- Phalanges
- Phalanges
- Ungual process

HINDLIMB

- Tibia
- Fibula
- Calcaneus
- Talus
- Tarsals
- Metatarsals
- Phalanges
- Ungual process

This Book Belongs To

Dog skull anatomy

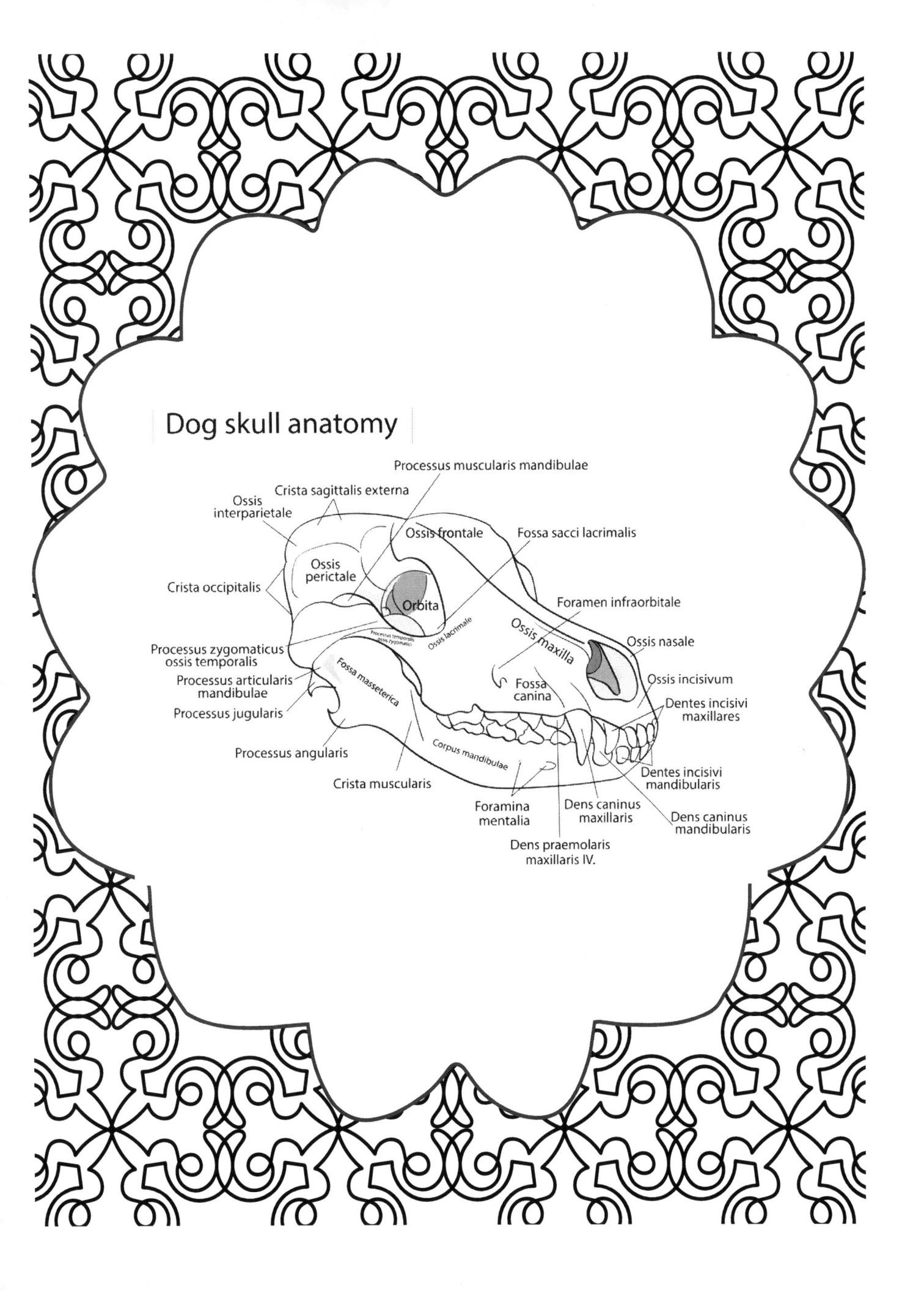

- Processus muscularis mandibulae
- Crista sagittalis externa
- Ossis interparietale
- Ossis frontale
- Fossa sacci lacrimalis
- Ossis perictale
- Crista occipitalis
- Orbita
- Foramen infraorbitale
- Processus temporalis ossis zygomatici
- Ossis lacrimale
- Ossis maxilla
- Ossis nasale
- Processus zygomaticus ossis temporalis
- Fossa masseterica
- Ossis incisivum
- Processus articularis mandibulae
- Fossa canina
- Dentes incisivi maxillares
- Processus jugularis
- Corpus mandibulae
- Dentes incisivi mandibularis
- Processus angularis
- Crista muscularis
- Dens caninus maxillaris
- Dens caninus mandibularis
- Foramina mentalia
- Dens praemolaris maxillaris IV.

Heart of the dog

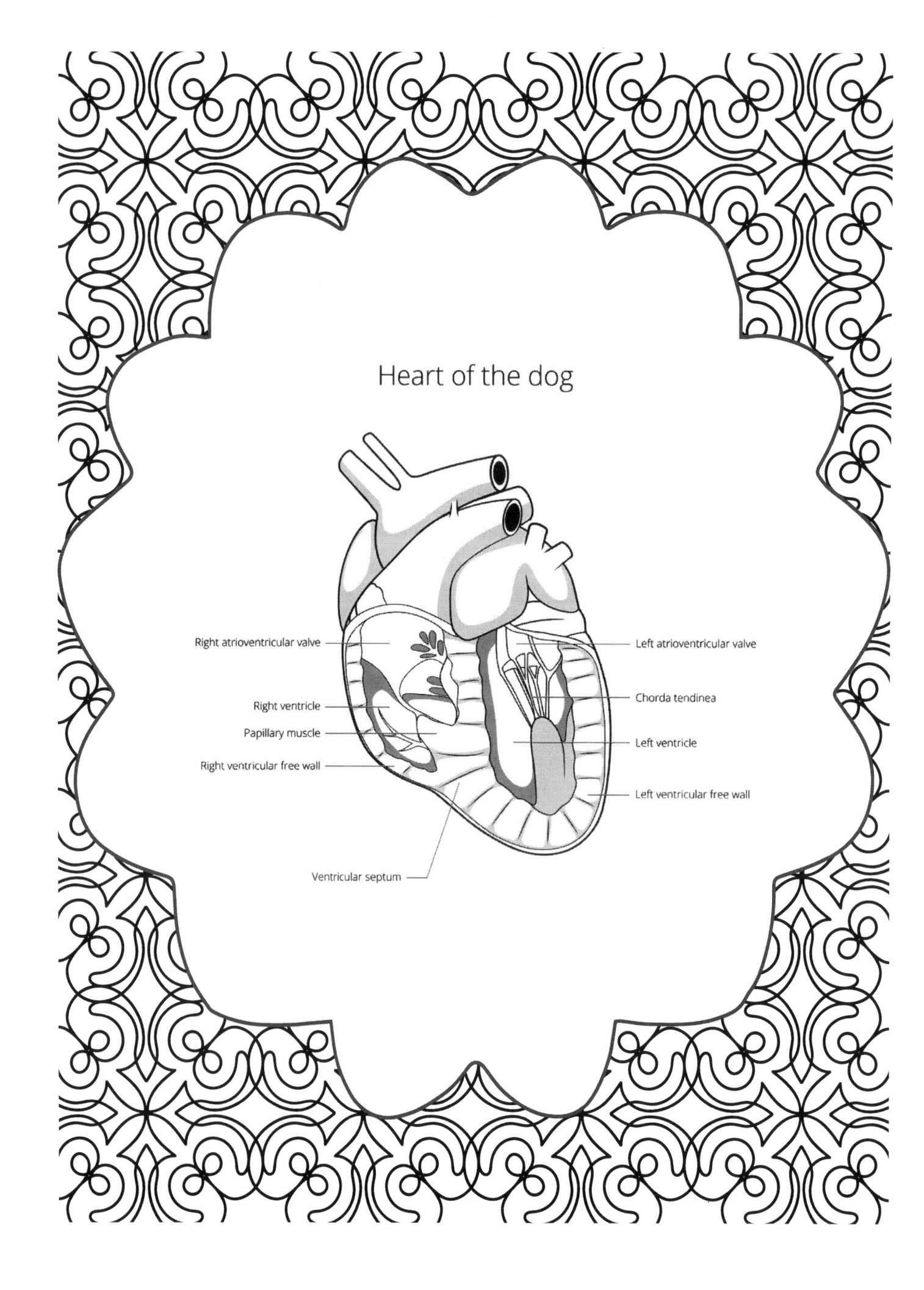

- Right atrioventricular valve
- Right ventricle
- Papillary muscle
- Right ventricular free wall
- Ventricular septum
- Left atrioventricular valve
- Chorda tendinea
- Left ventricle
- Left ventricular free wall

Back skull

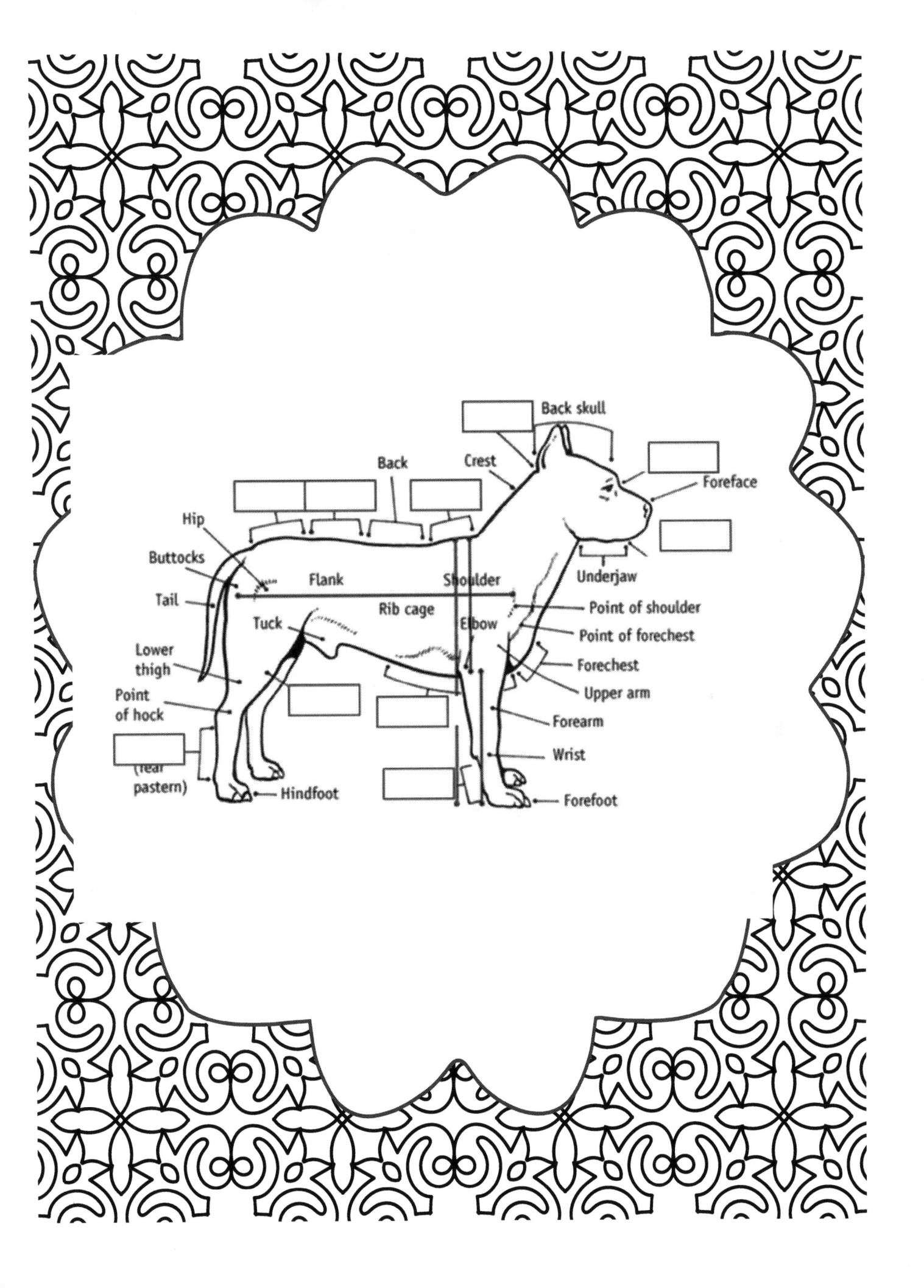

Back

Crest

Foreface

Hip

Buttocks

Underjaw

Tail

Flank

Shoulder

Point of shoulder

Rib cage

Tuck

Elbow

Point of forechest

Lower thigh

Forechest

Point of hock

Upper arm

Forearm

(rear pastern)

Wrist

Hindfoot

Forefoot

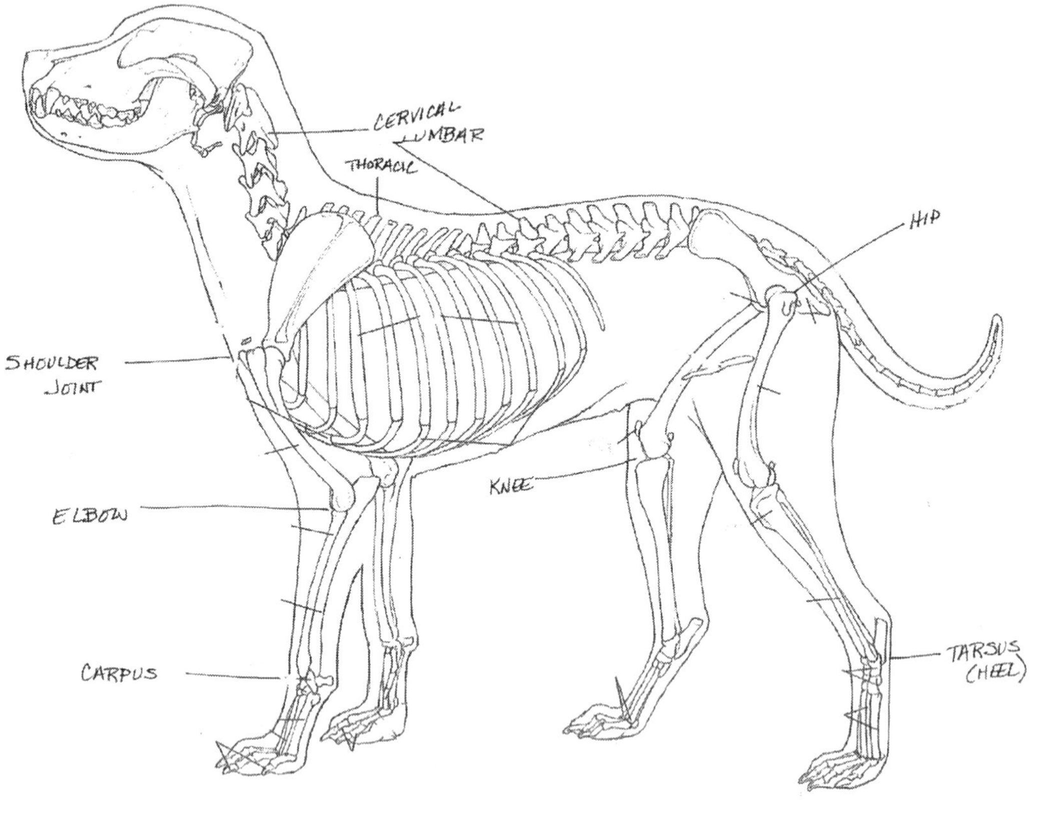
CERVICAL
LUMBAR
THORACIC
HIP
SHOULDER JOINT
ELBOW
KNEE
CARPUS
TARSUS (HEEL)

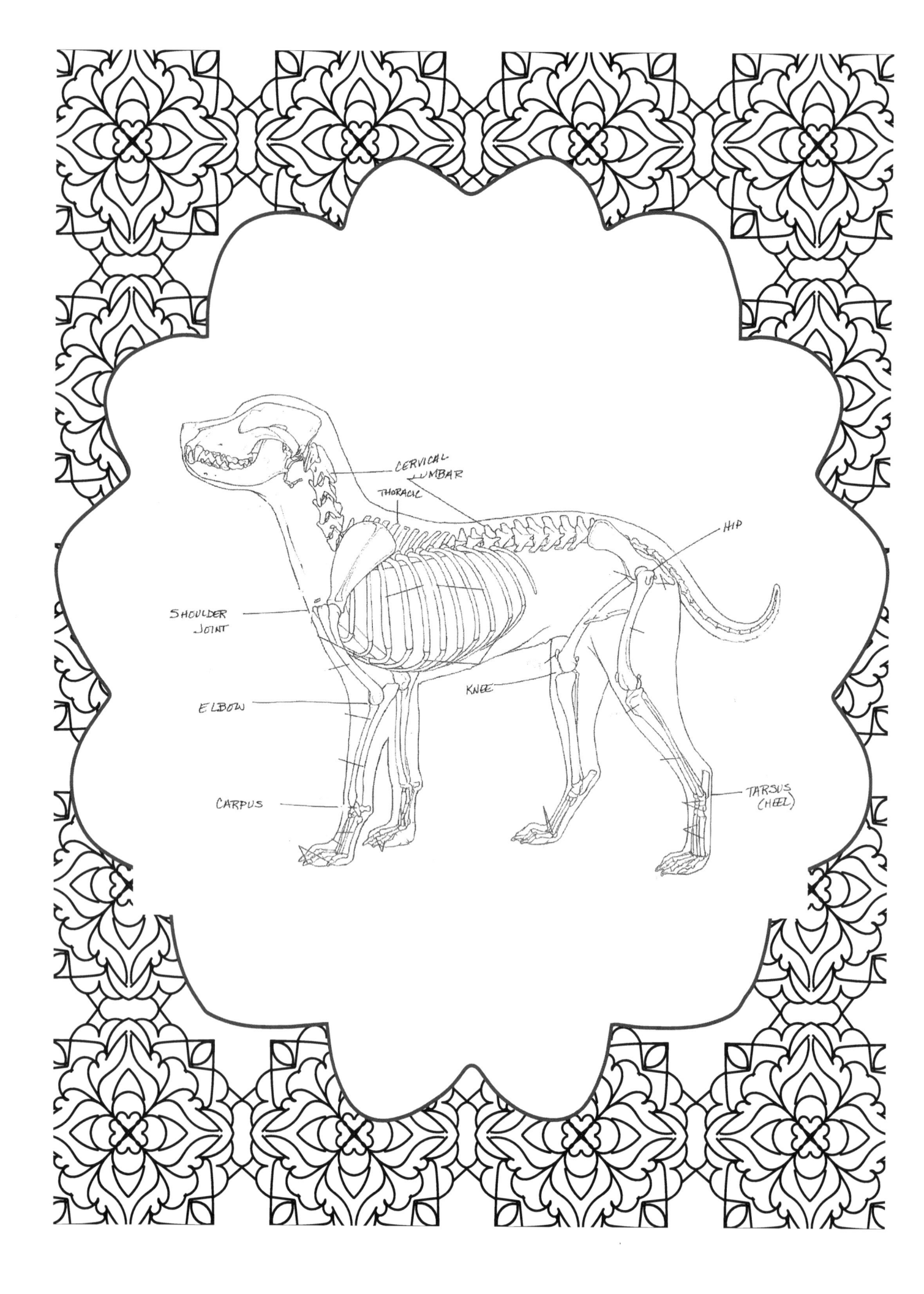

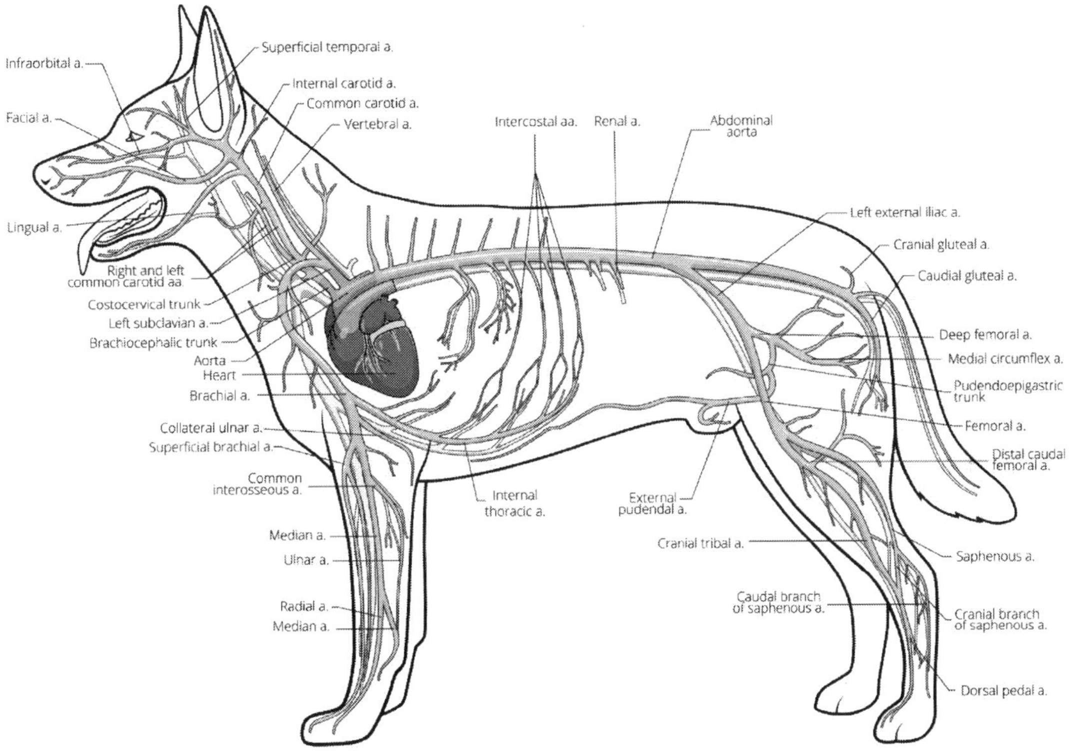

Infraorbital a.
Superficial temporal a.
Internal carotid a.
Common carotid a.
Vertebral a.
Facial a.
Intercostal aa.
Renal a.
Abdominal aorta
Lingual a.
Left external iliac a.
Cranial gluteal a.
Right and left common carotid aa
Caudial gluteal a.
Costocervical trunk
Left subclavian a.
Brachiocephalic trunk
Deep femoral a.
Aorta
Medial circumflex a.
Heart
Pudendoepigastric trunk
Brachial a.
Femoral a.
Collateral ulnar a.
Superficial brachial a.
Distal caudal femoral a.
Common interosseous a.
Internal thoracic a.
External pudendal a.
Median a.
Cranial tribal a.
Saphenous a.
Ulnar a.
Caudal branch of saphenous a.
Radial a.
Cranial branch of saphenous a.
Median a.
Dorsal pedal a.

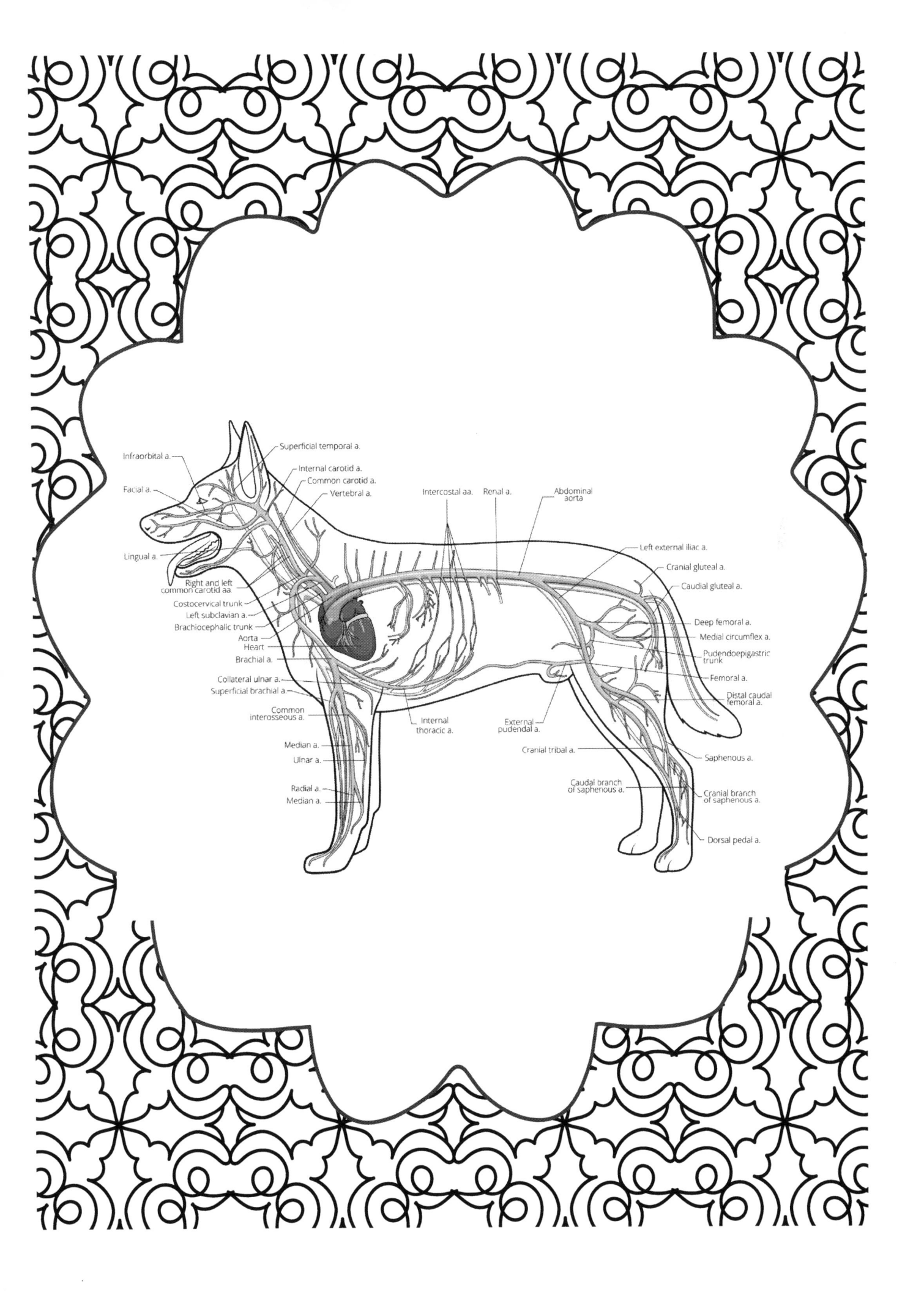

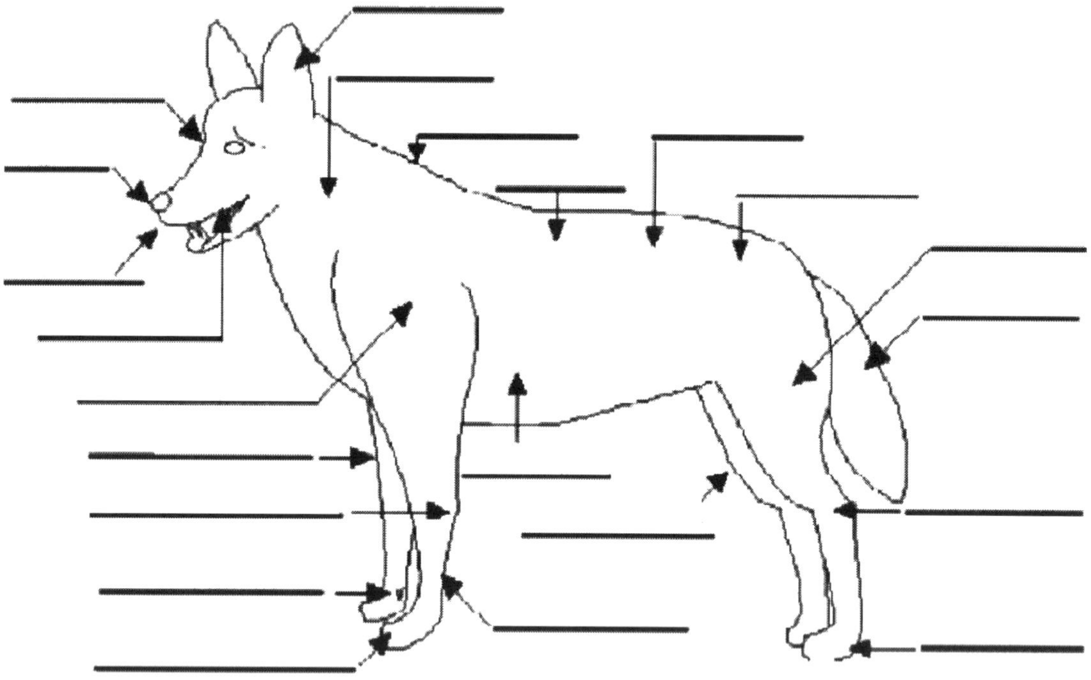

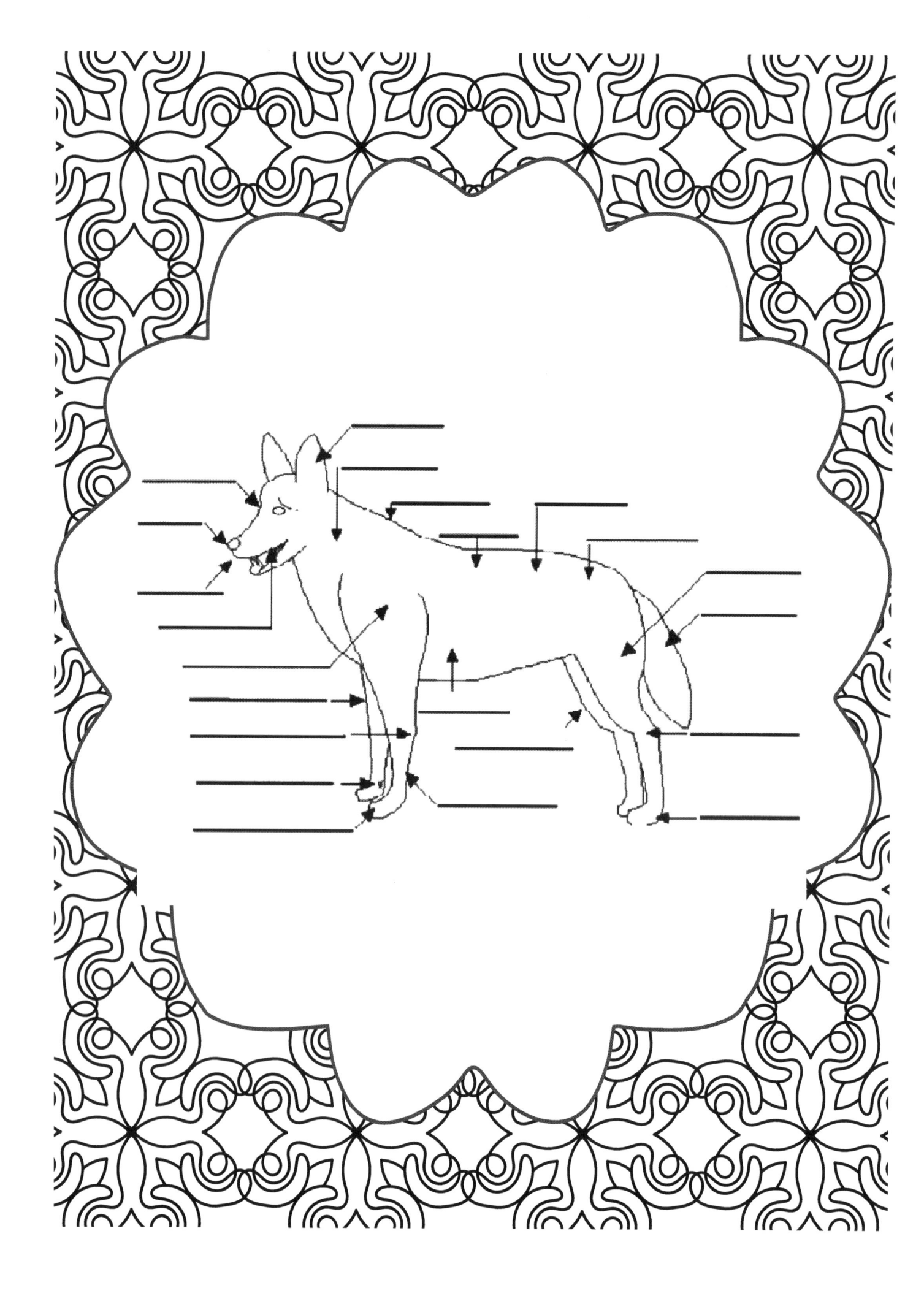

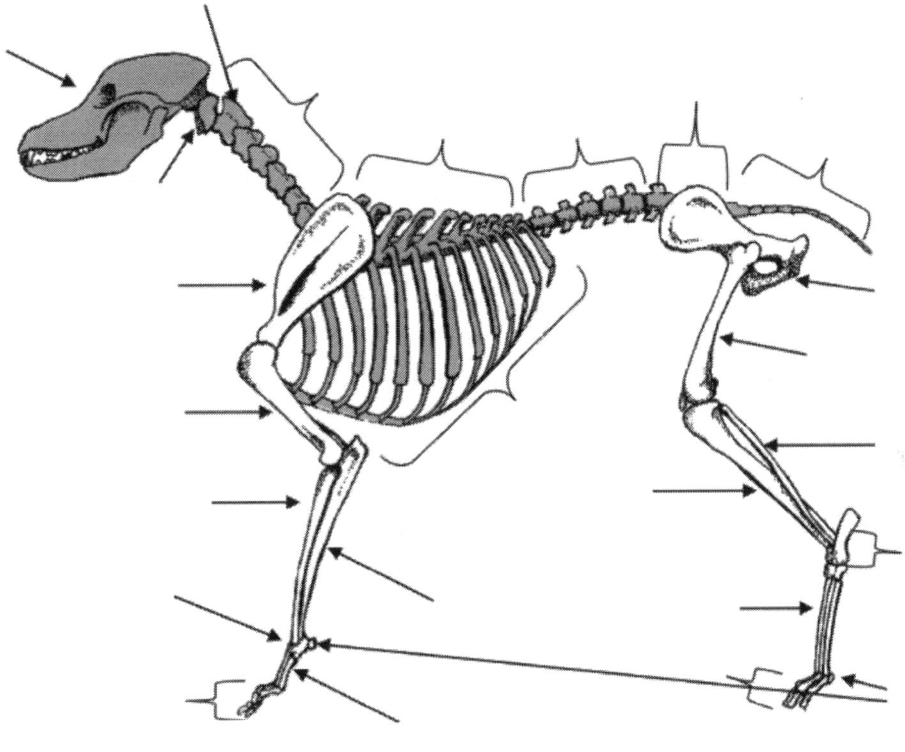

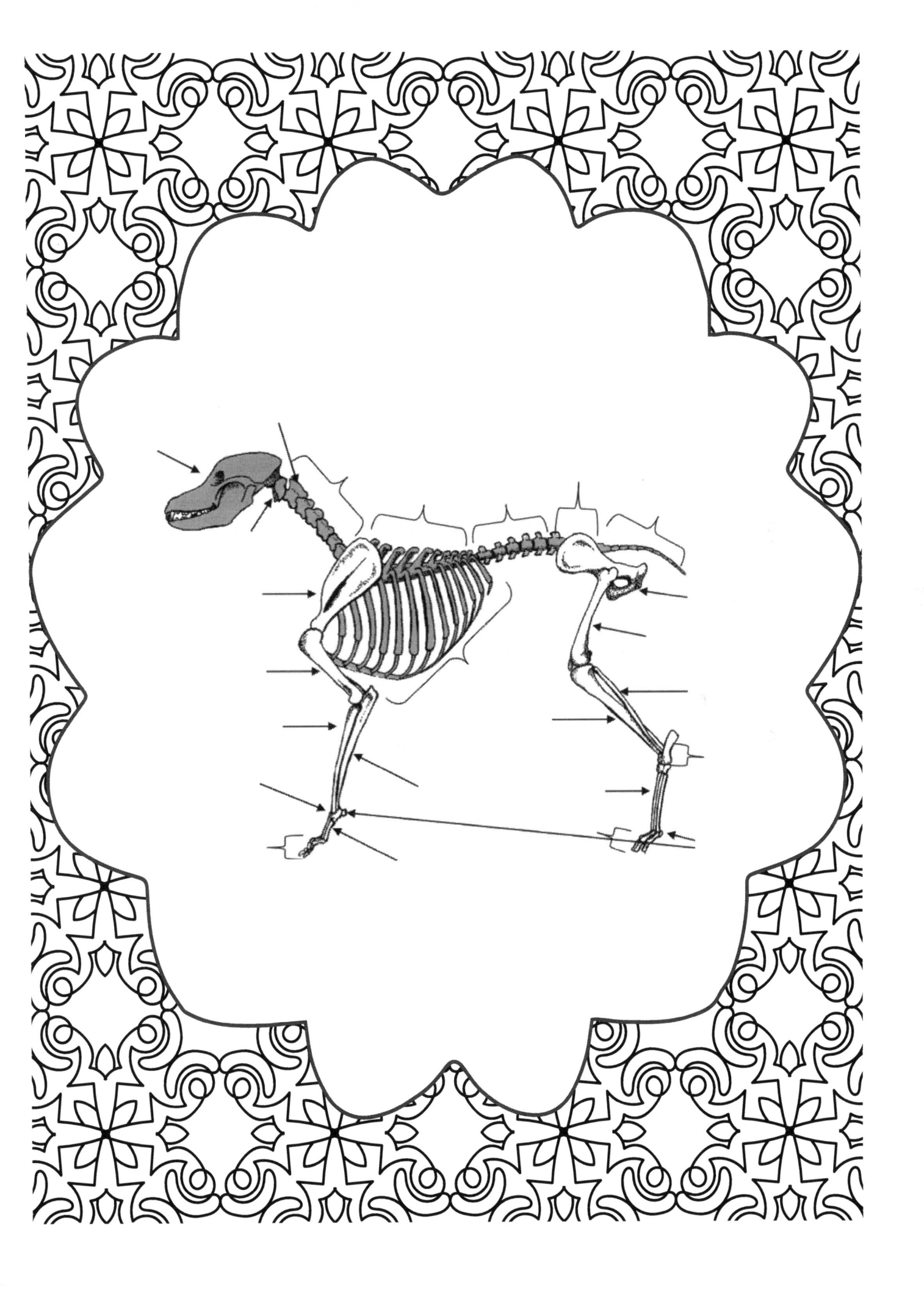

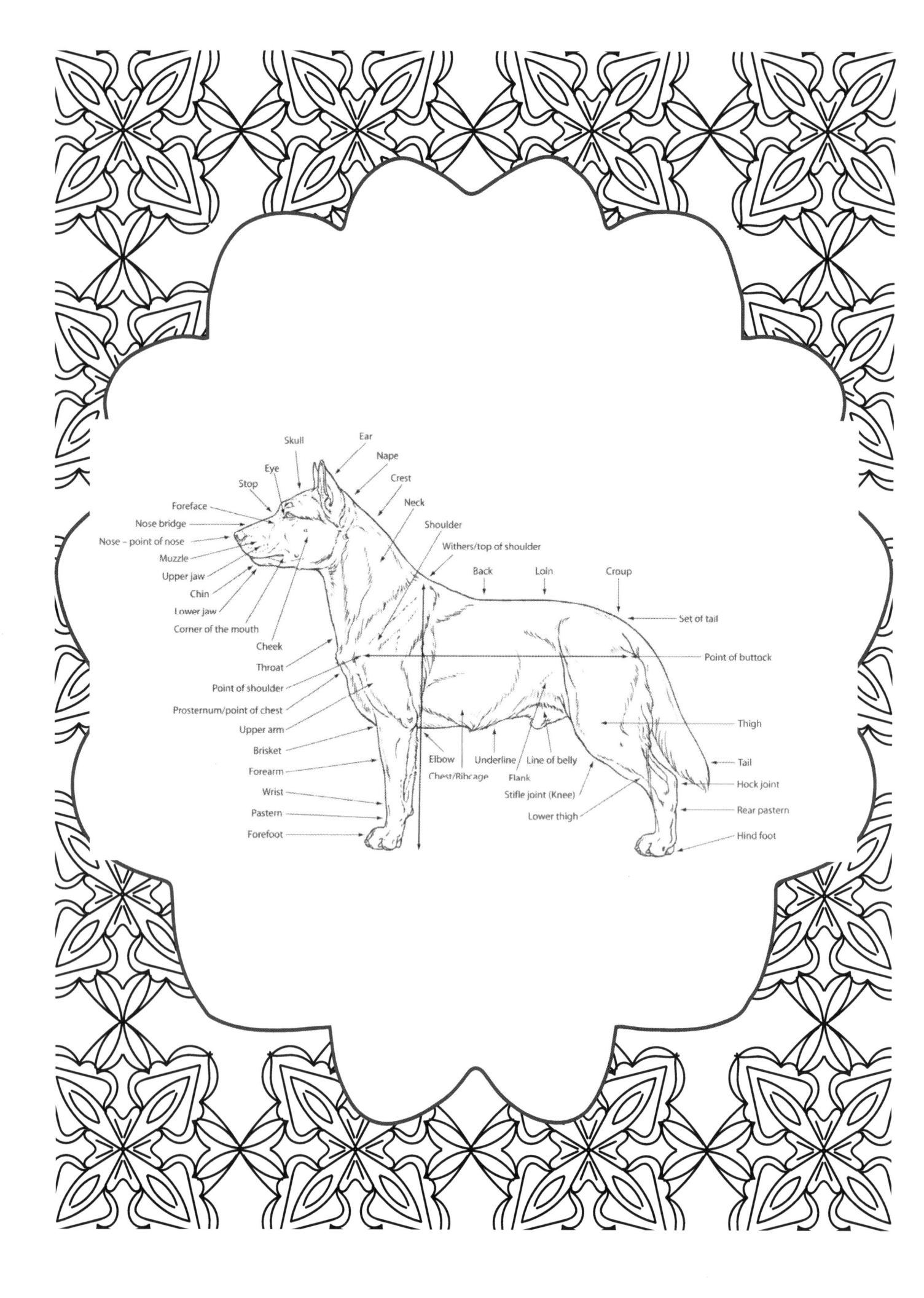

Skull
Ear
Eye
Nape
Stop
Crest
Foreface
Neck
Nose bridge
Shoulder
Nose – point of nose
Withers/top of shoulder
Muzzle
Back
Loin
Croup
Upper jaw
Chin
Set of tail
Lower jaw
Corner of the mouth
Point of buttock
Cheek
Throat
Point of shoulder
Prosternum/point of chest
Thigh
Upper arm
Brisket
Tail
Forearm
Elbow
Underline
Line of belly
Hock joint
Wrist
Chest/Ribcage
Flank
Pastern
Stifle joint (Knee)
Rear pastern
Lower thigh
Forefoot
Hind foot

ANATOMY OF A DOG

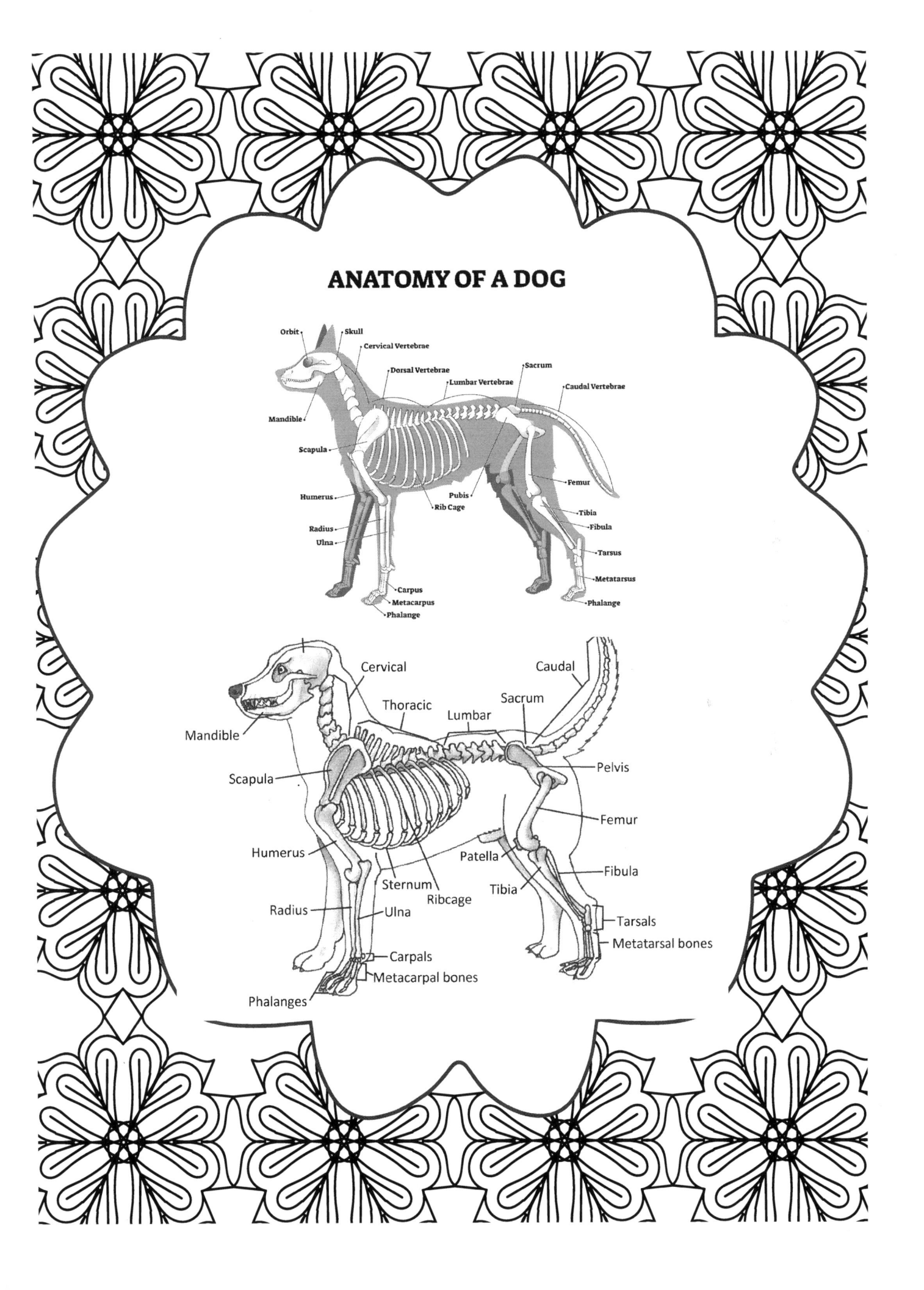

ANATOMY OF THE DIGESTIVE SYSTEM

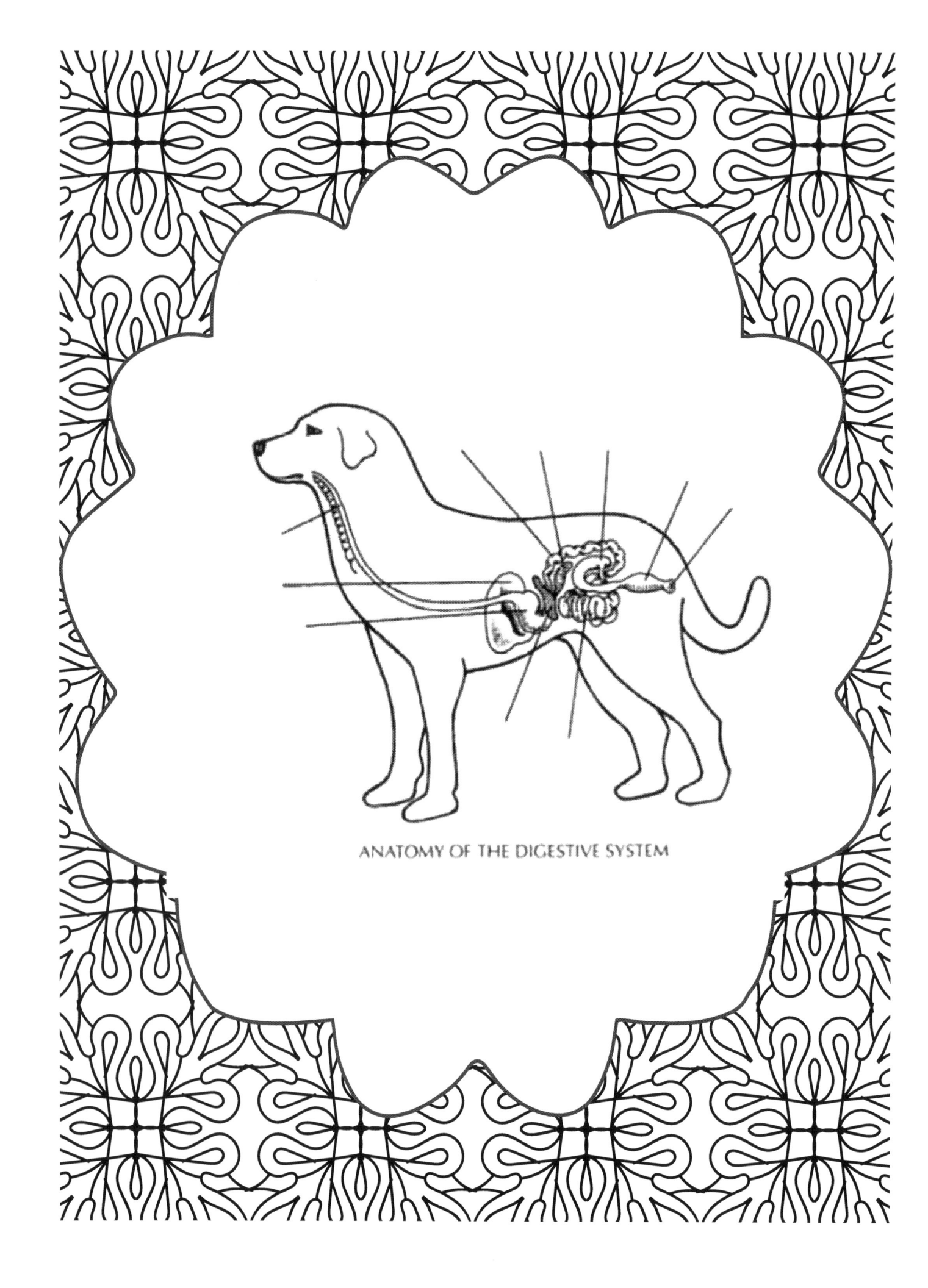

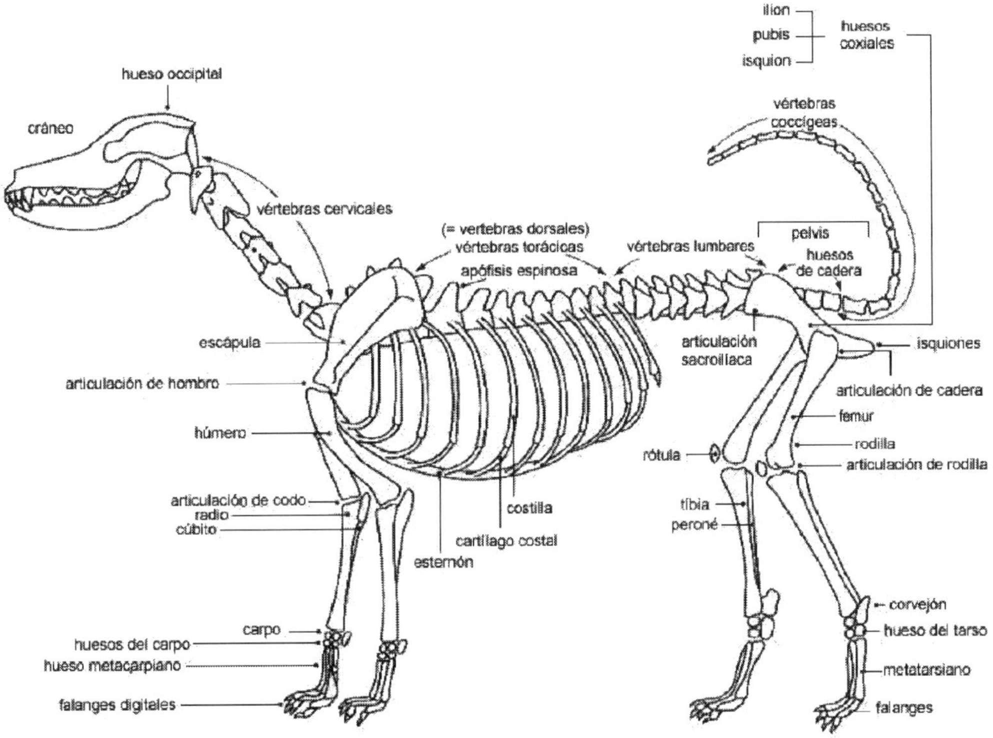
ilion
pubis
isquion
huesos coxiales
hueso occipital
cráneo
vértebras coccígeas
vértebras cervicales
(= vertebras dorsales)
vértebras torácicas
pelvis
vértebras lumbares
huesos de cadera
apófisis espinosa
escápula
articulación sacroilíaca
isquiones
articulación de hombro
articulación de cadera
fémur
húmero
rodilla
rótula
articulación de rodilla
articulación de codo
radio
cúbito
costilla
tibia
peroné
cartílago costal
esternón
corvejón
carpo
hueso del tarso
huesos del carpo
hueso metacarpiano
metatarsiano
falanges digitales
falanges

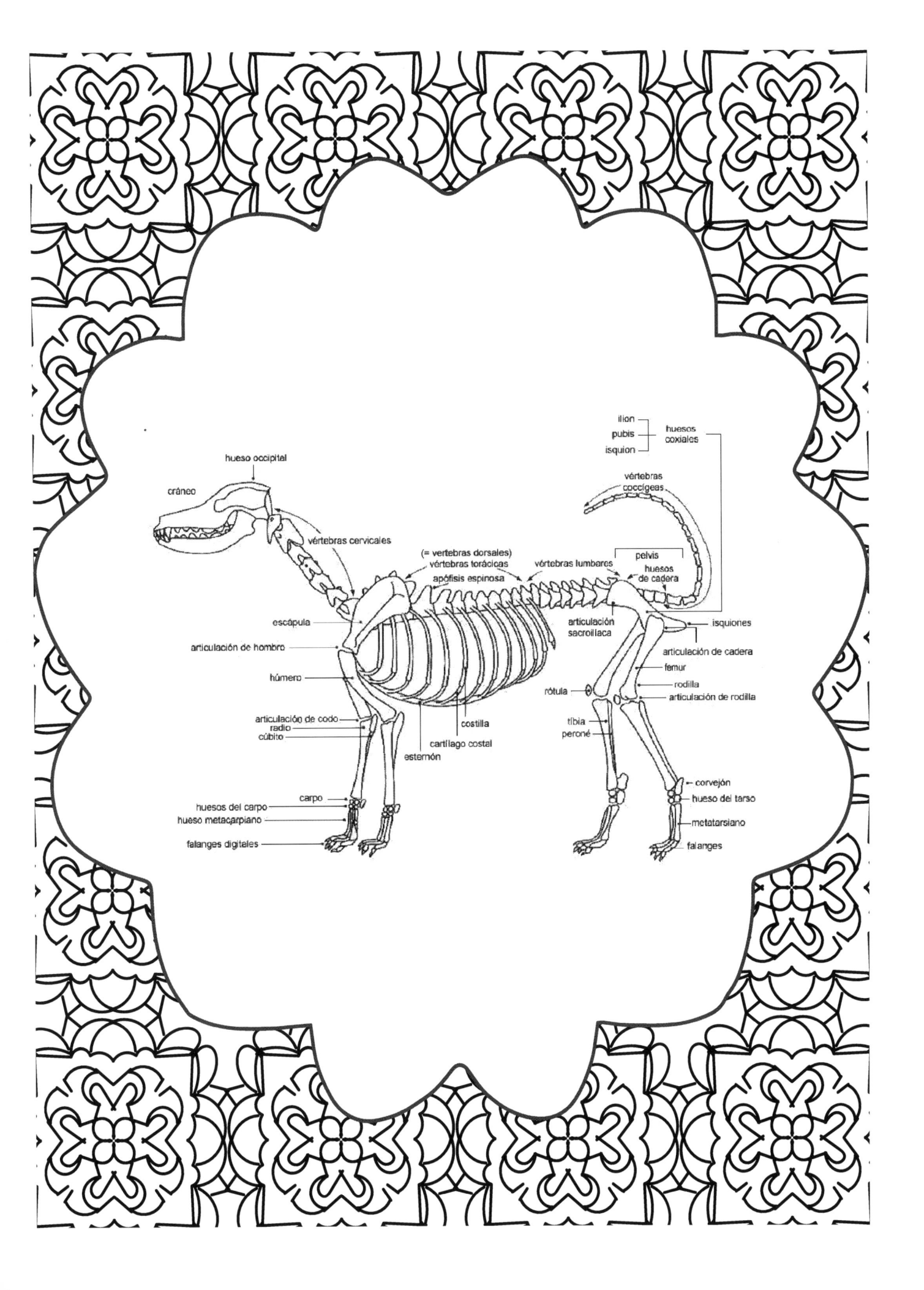

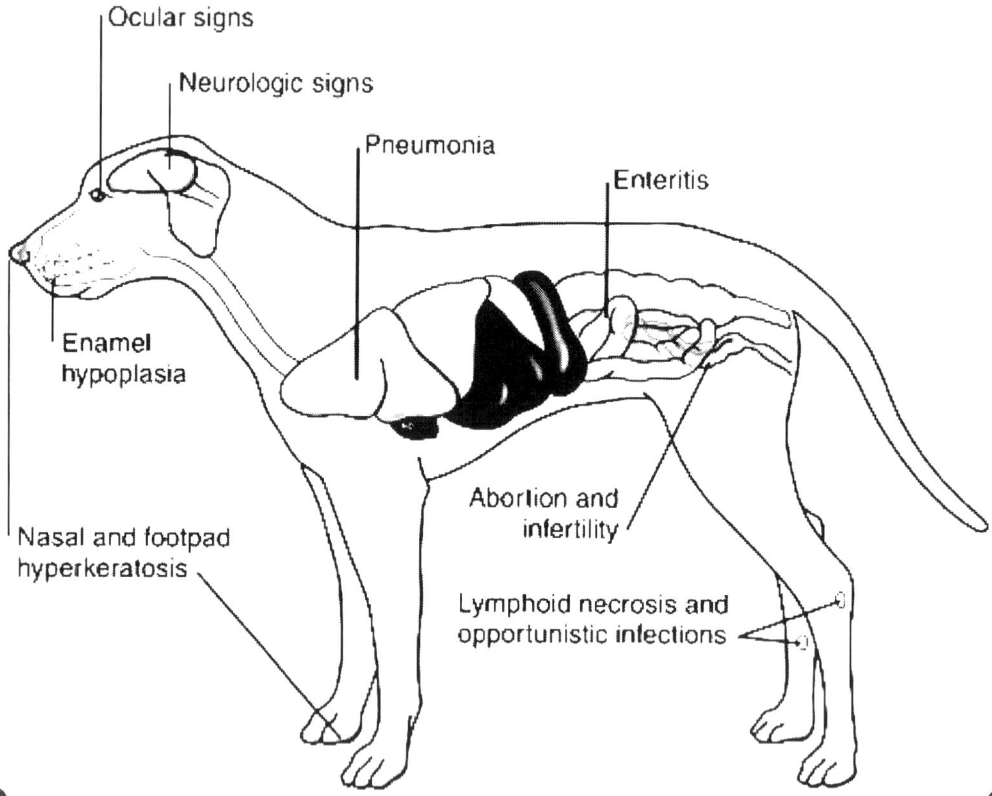
Ocular signs
Neurologic signs
Pneumonia
Enteritis
Enamel
hypoplasia
Abortion and
infertility
Nasal and footpad
hyperkeratosis
Lymphoid necrosis and
opportunistic infections

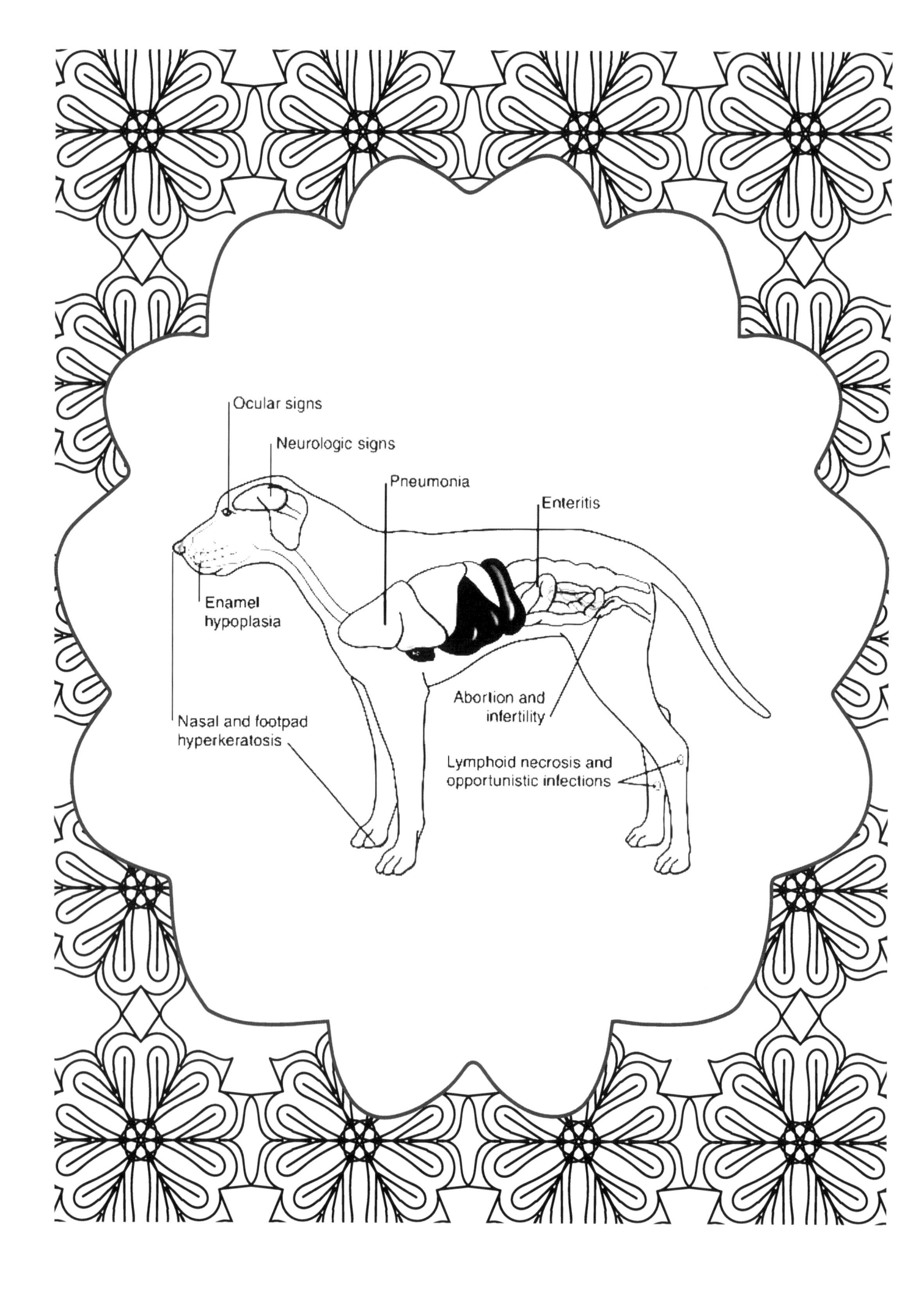

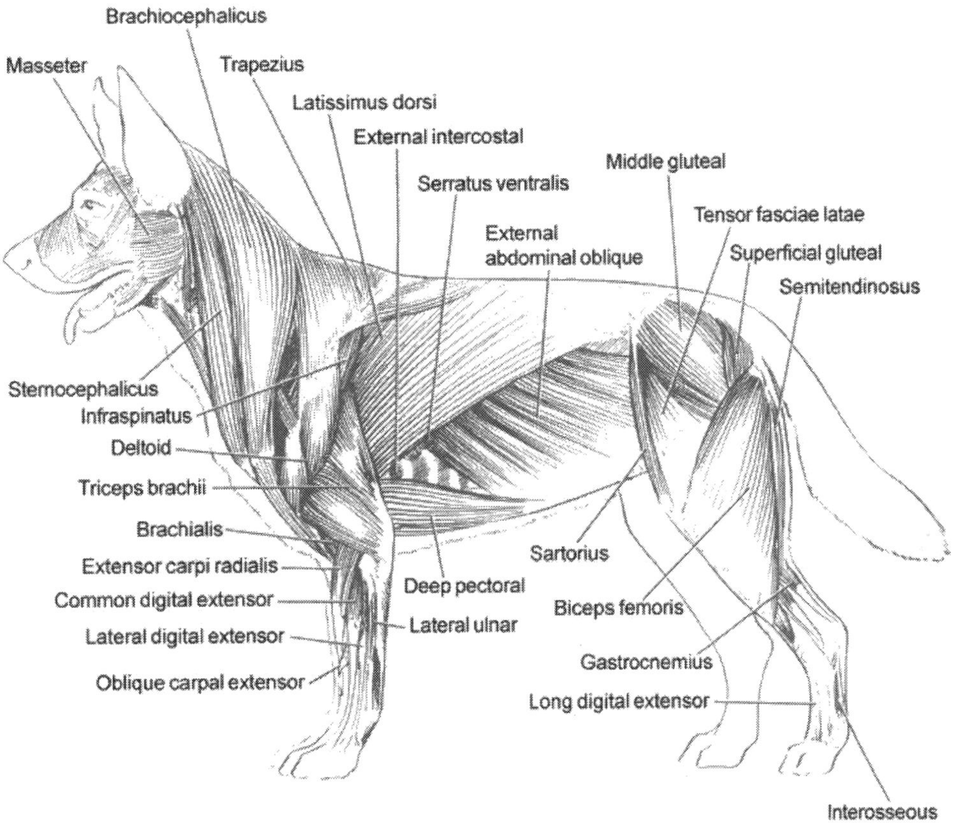
Brachiocephalicus
Masseter
Trapezius
Latissimus dorsi
External intercostal
Serratus ventralis
Middle gluteal
Tensor fasciae latae
External
abdominal oblique
Superficial gluteal
Semitendinosus
Sternocephalicus
Infraspinatus
Deltoid
Triceps brachii
Brachialis
Extensor carpi radialis
Common digital extensor
Lateral digital extensor
Oblique carpal extensor
Deep pectoral
Lateral ulnar
Sartorius
Biceps femoris
Gastrocnemius
Long digital extensor
Interosseous

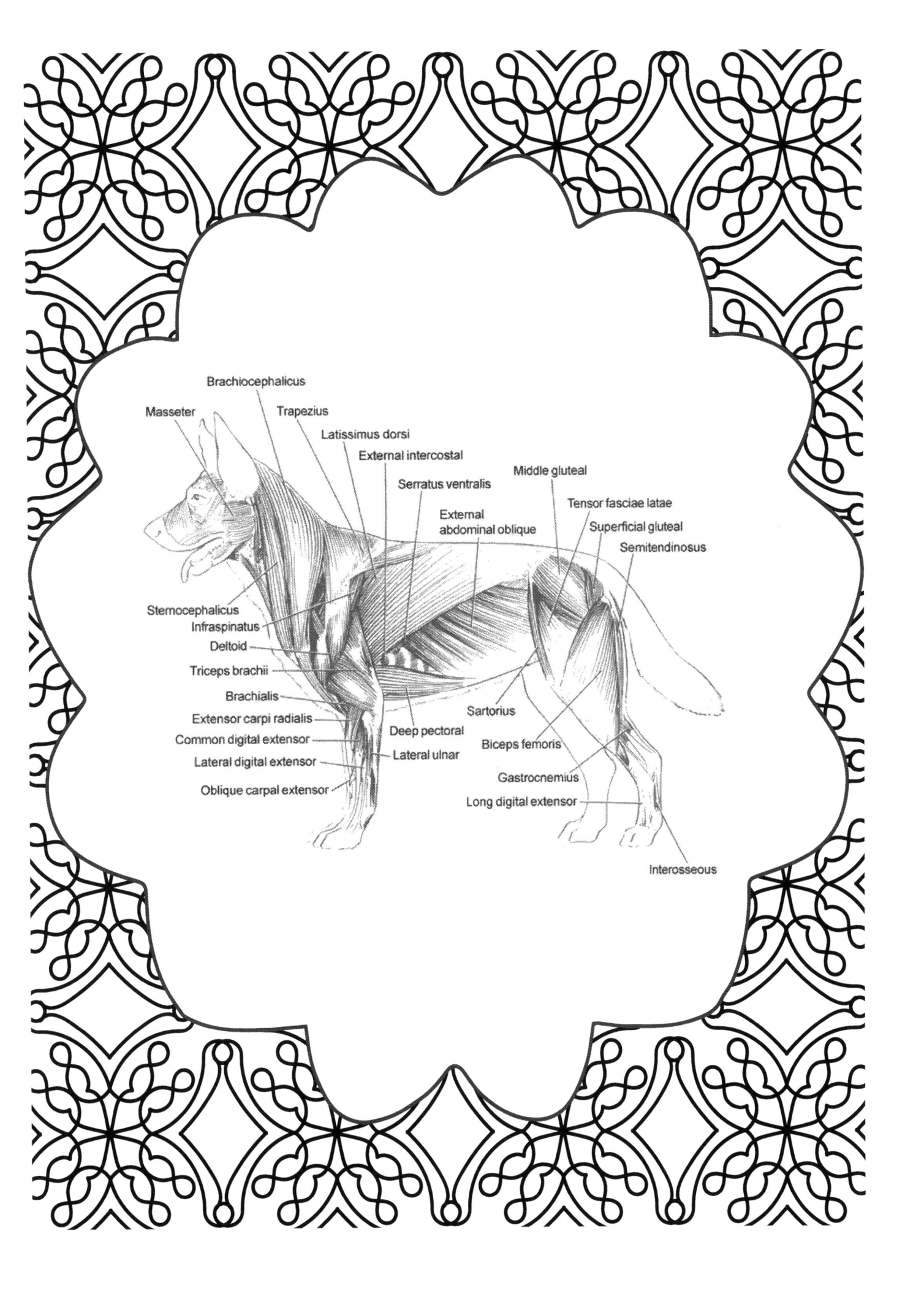

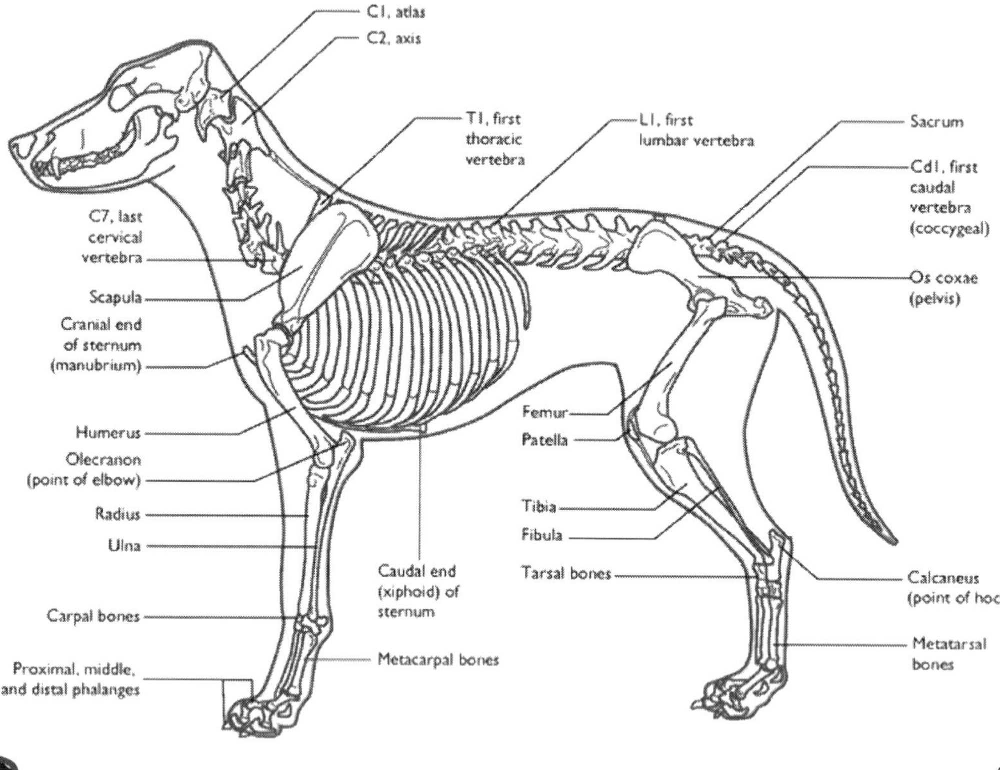

C1, atlas
C2, axis
T1, first thoracic vertebra
L1, first lumbar vertebra
Sacrum
Cd1, first caudal vertebra (coccygeal)
C7, last cervical vertebra
Scapula
Os coxae (pelvis)
Cranial end of sternum (manubrium)
Femur
Patella
Humerus
Olecranon (point of elbow)
Tibia
Radius
Fibula
Ulna
Caudal end (xiphoid) of sternum
Tarsal bones
Calcaneus (point of hock)
Carpal bones
Metacarpal bones
Metatarsal bones
Proximal, middle, and distal phalanges

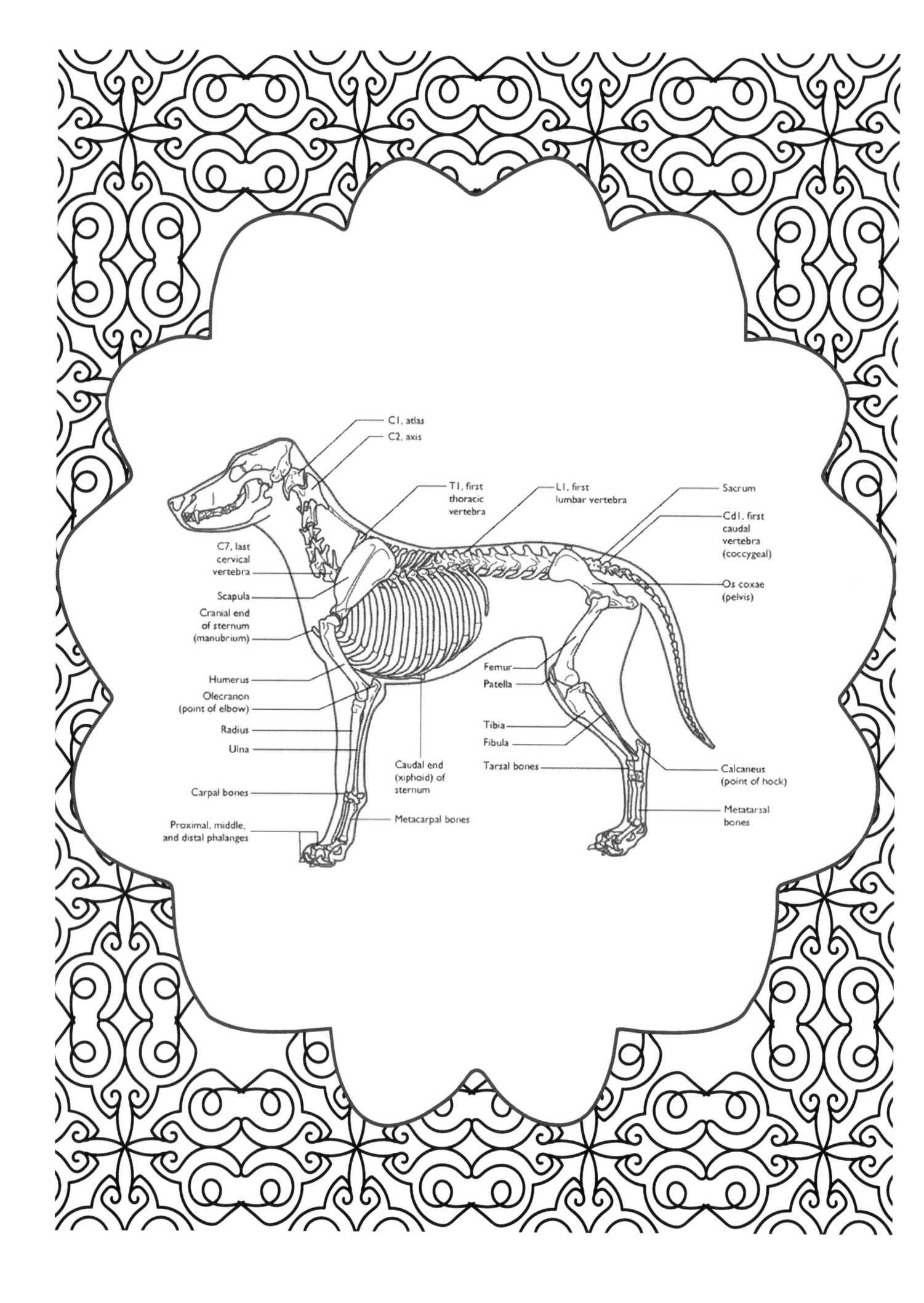

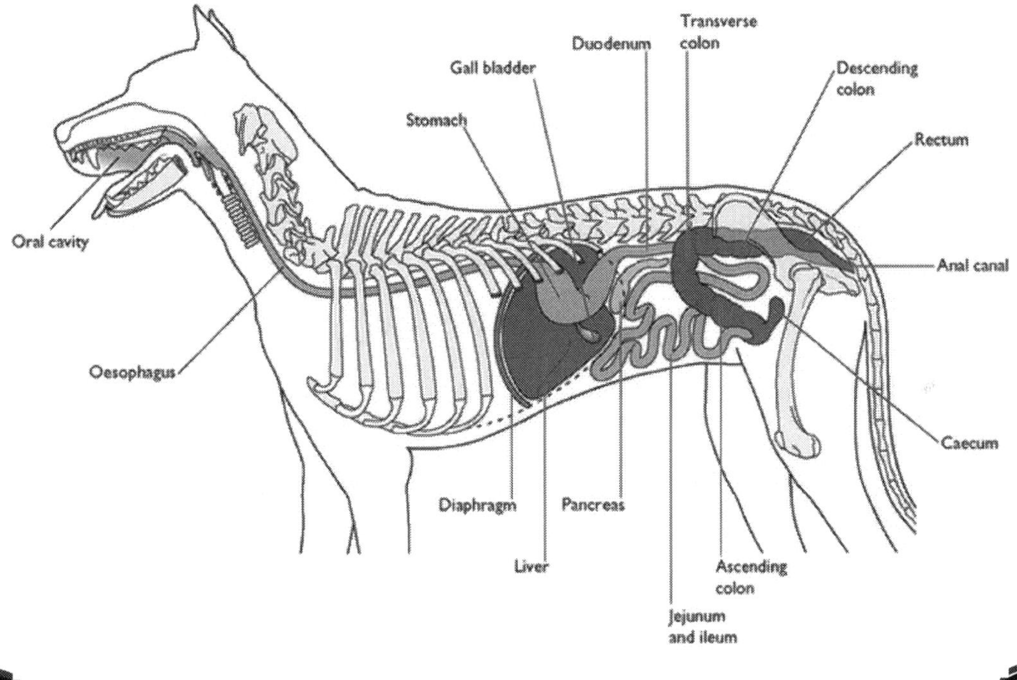
Transverse
colon
Duodenum
Gall bladder
Descending
colon
Stomach
Rectum
Oral cavity
Anal canal
Oesophagus
Caecum
Diaphragm
Pancreas
Liver
Ascending
colon
Jejunum
and ileum

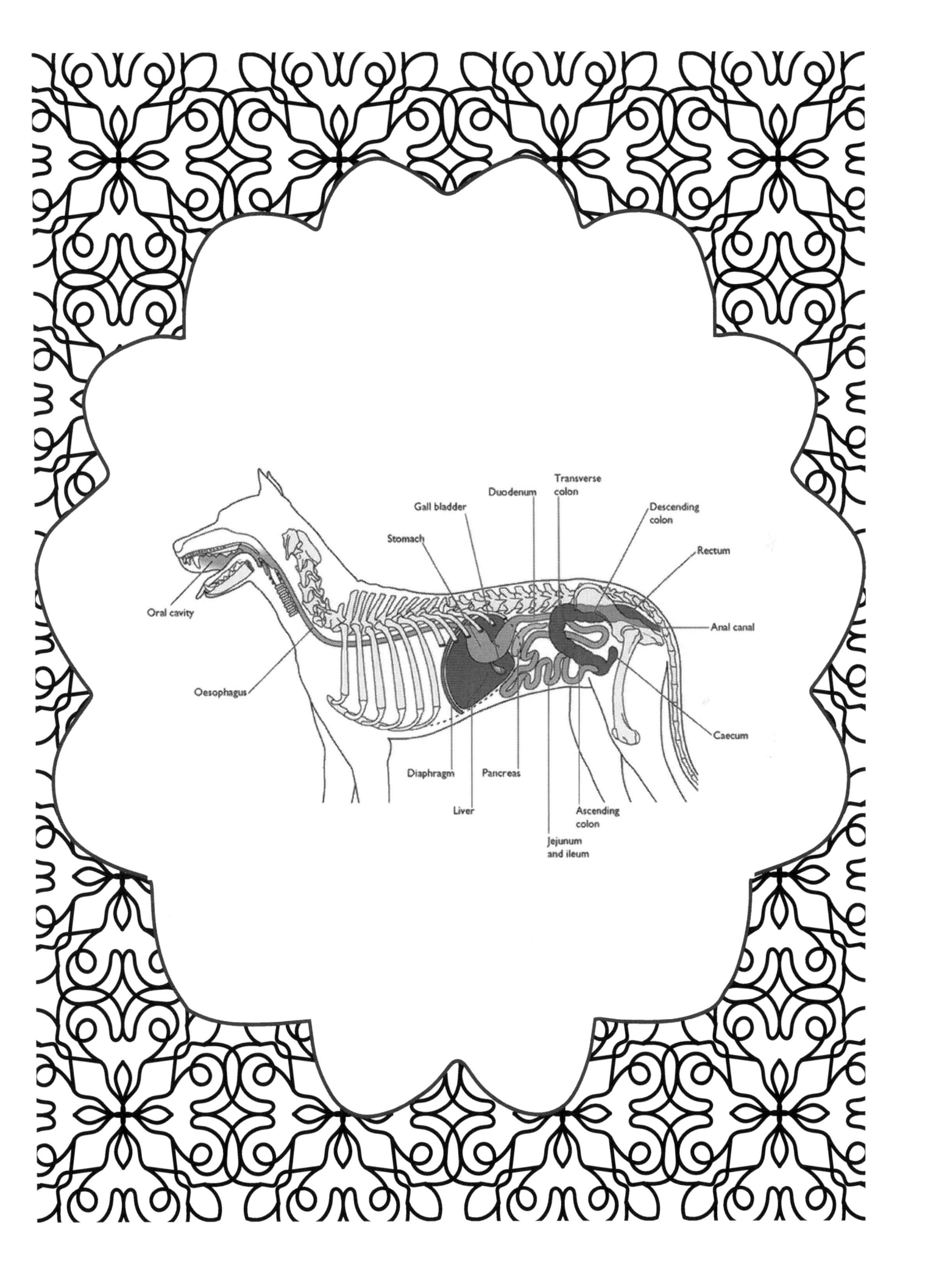

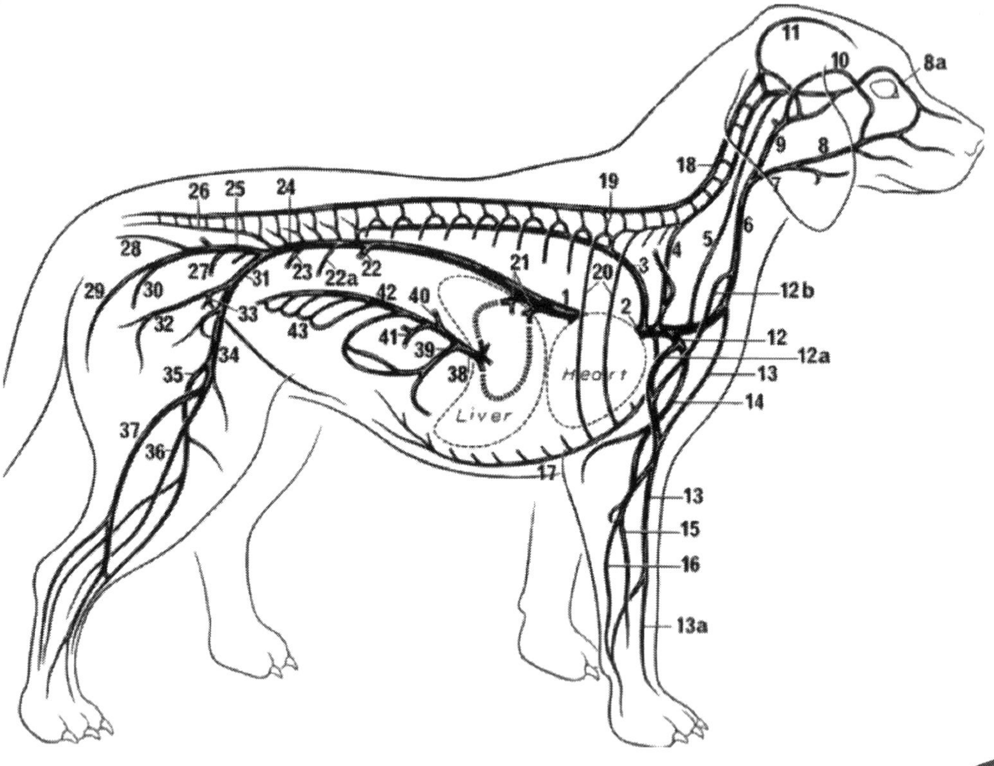

11
10
8a
9
8
7
18
19
6
5
4
3
26
25
24
28
27
23
22a
22
21
20
2
1
12b
29
30
31
33
42
40
32
43
41
39
12
12a
35
34
38
Heart
13
14
Liver
37
36
17
13
15
16
13a

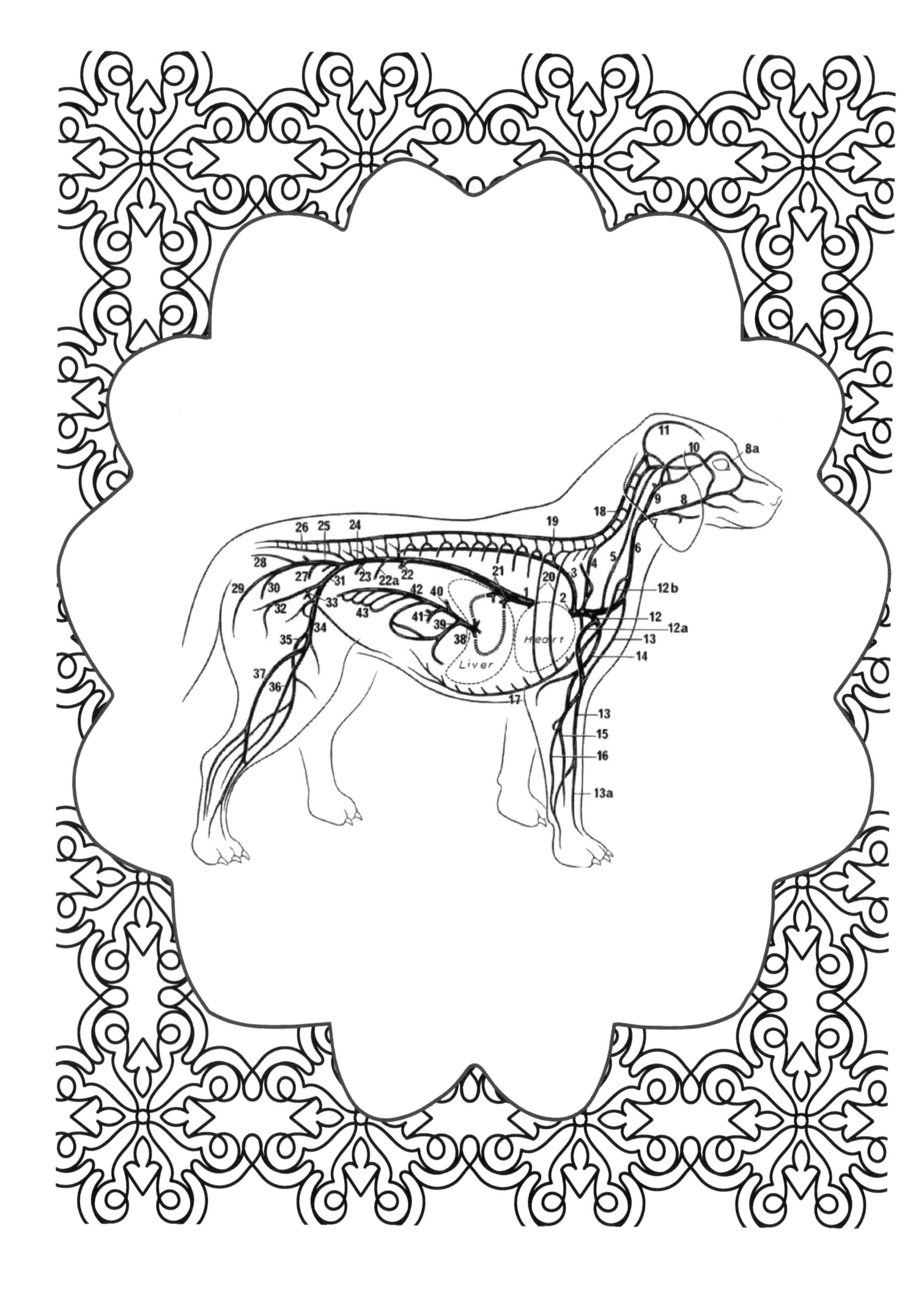

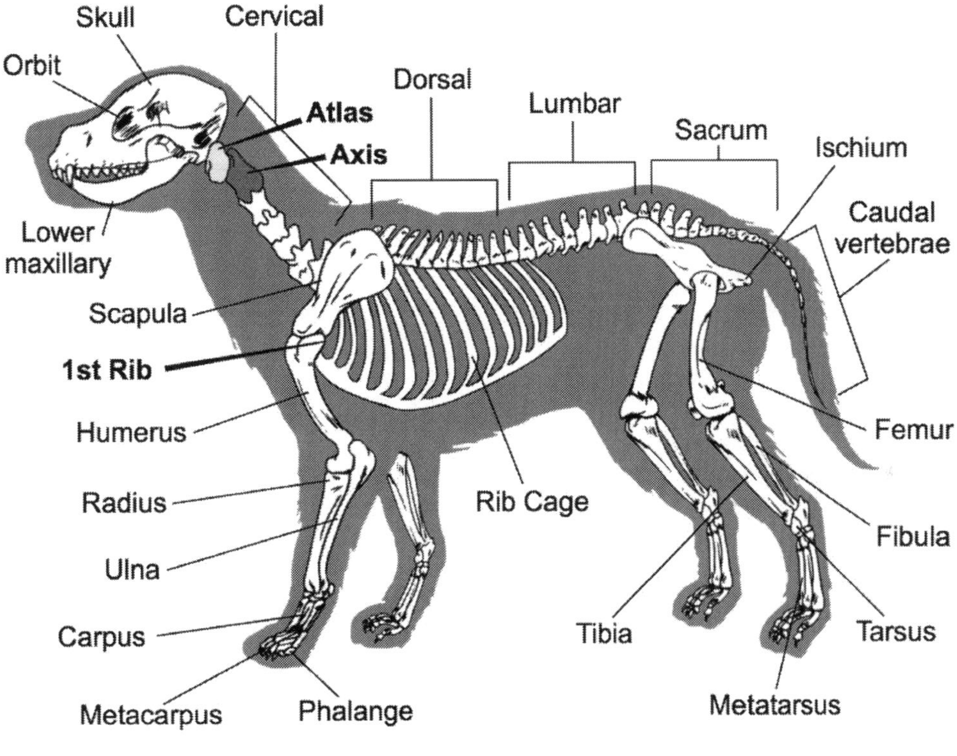

Skull
Cervical
Orbit
Dorsal
Lumbar
Atlas
Sacrum
Ischium
Axis
Caudal vertebrae
Lower maxillary
Scapula
1st Rib
Humerus
Femur
Radius
Rib Cage
Fibula
Ulna
Carpus
Tibia
Tarsus
Metacarpus
Phalange
Metatarsus

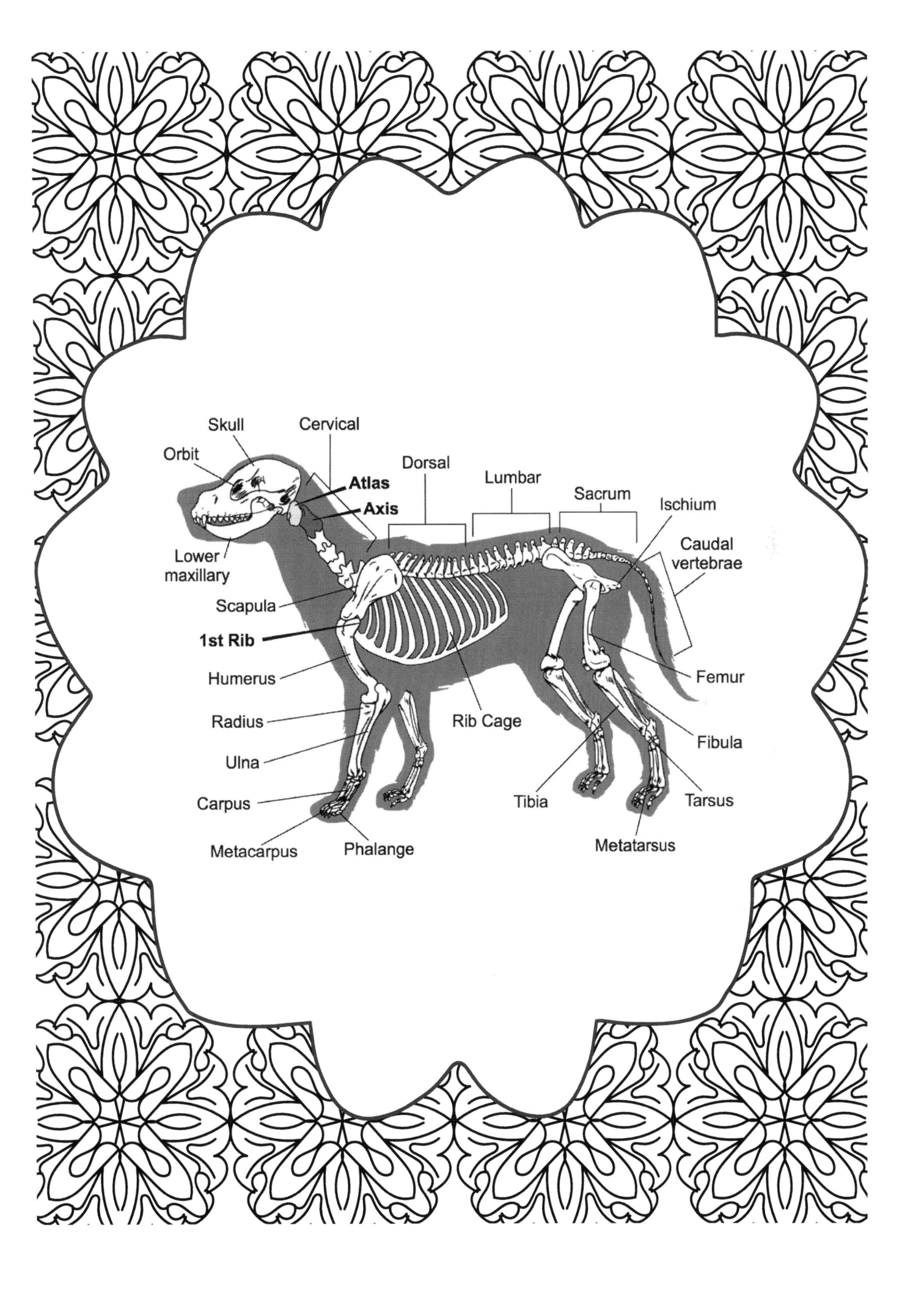

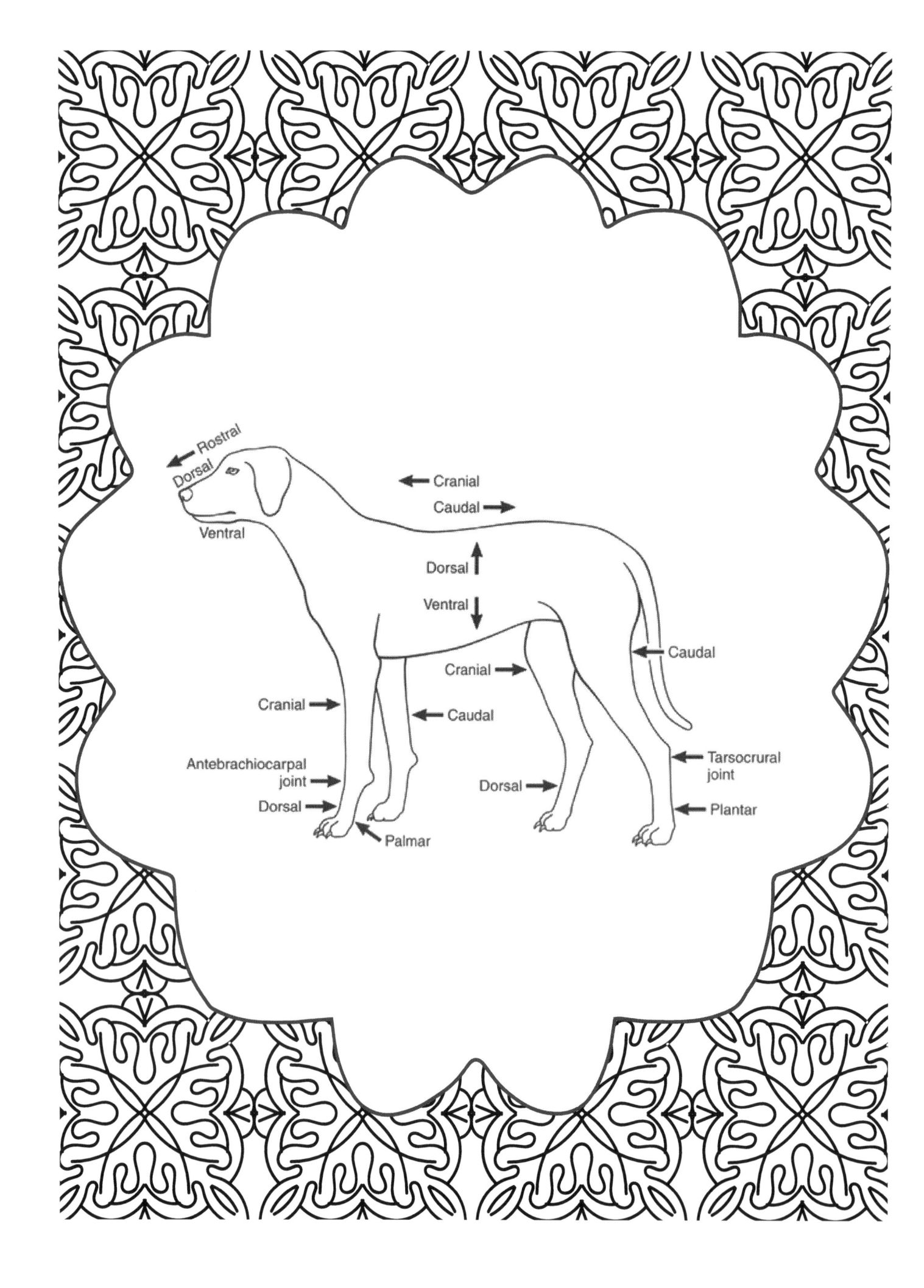

- Rostral
- Dorsal
- Ventral
- Cranial
- Caudal
- Dorsal
- Ventral
- Caudal
- Cranial
- Cranial
- Caudal
- Antebrachiocarpal joint
- Dorsal
- Palmar
- Dorsal
- Tarsocrural joint
- Plantar

Skeletal System

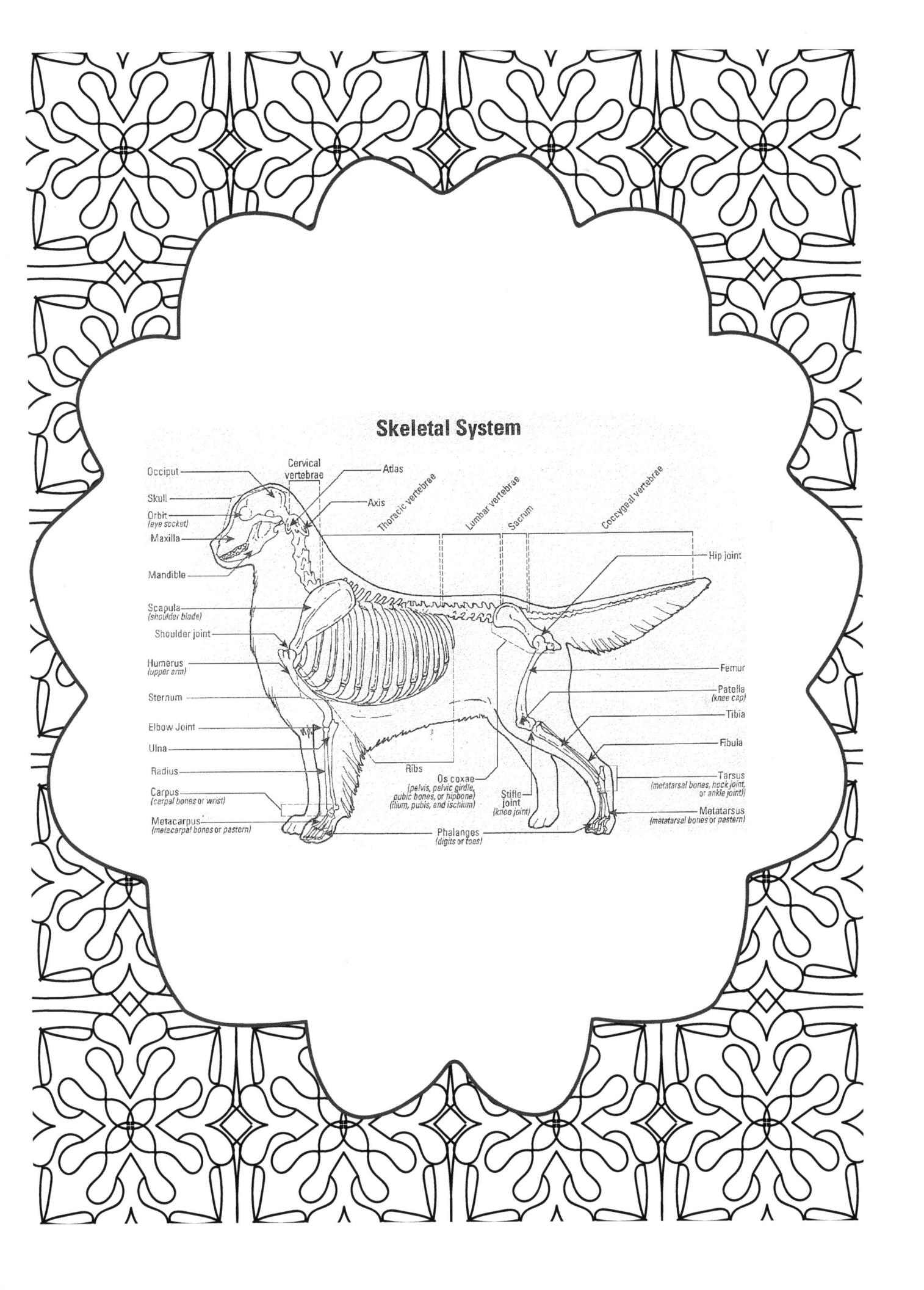

- Occiput
- Cervical vertebrae
- Atlas
- Skull
- Axis
- Thoracic vertebrae
- Lumbar vertebrae
- Sacrum
- Coccygeal vertebrae
- Orbit (eye socket)
- Maxilla
- Hip joint
- Mandible
- Scapula (shoulder blade)
- Shoulder joint
- Femur
- Humerus (upper arm)
- Patella (knee cap)
- Sternum
- Tibia
- Elbow Joint
- Fibula
- Ulna
- Radius
- Ribs
- Tarsus (metatarsal bones, hock joint, or ankle joint)
- Carpus (carpal bones or wrist)
- Os coxae (pelvis, pelvic girdle, pubic bones, or hipbone) (ilium, pubis, and ischium)
- Stifle joint (knee joint)
- Metacarpus (metacarpal bones or pastern)
- Metatarsus (metatarsal bones or pastern)
- Phalanges (digits or toes)

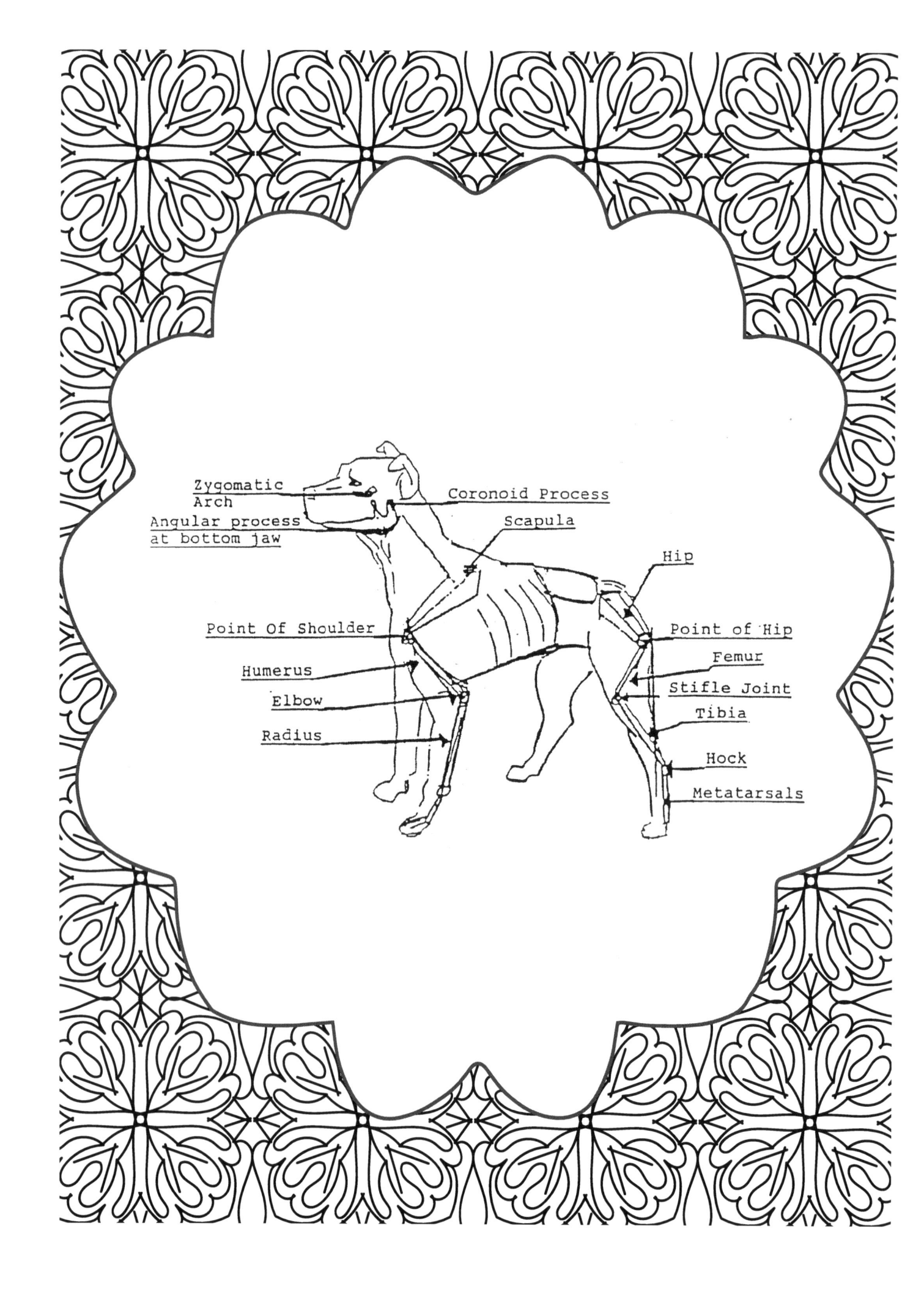

Zygomatic Arch
Coronoid Process
Angular process at bottom jaw
Scapula
Hip
Point Of Shoulder
Point of Hip
Humerus
Femur
Elbow
Stifle Joint
Radius
Tibia
Hock
Metatarsals

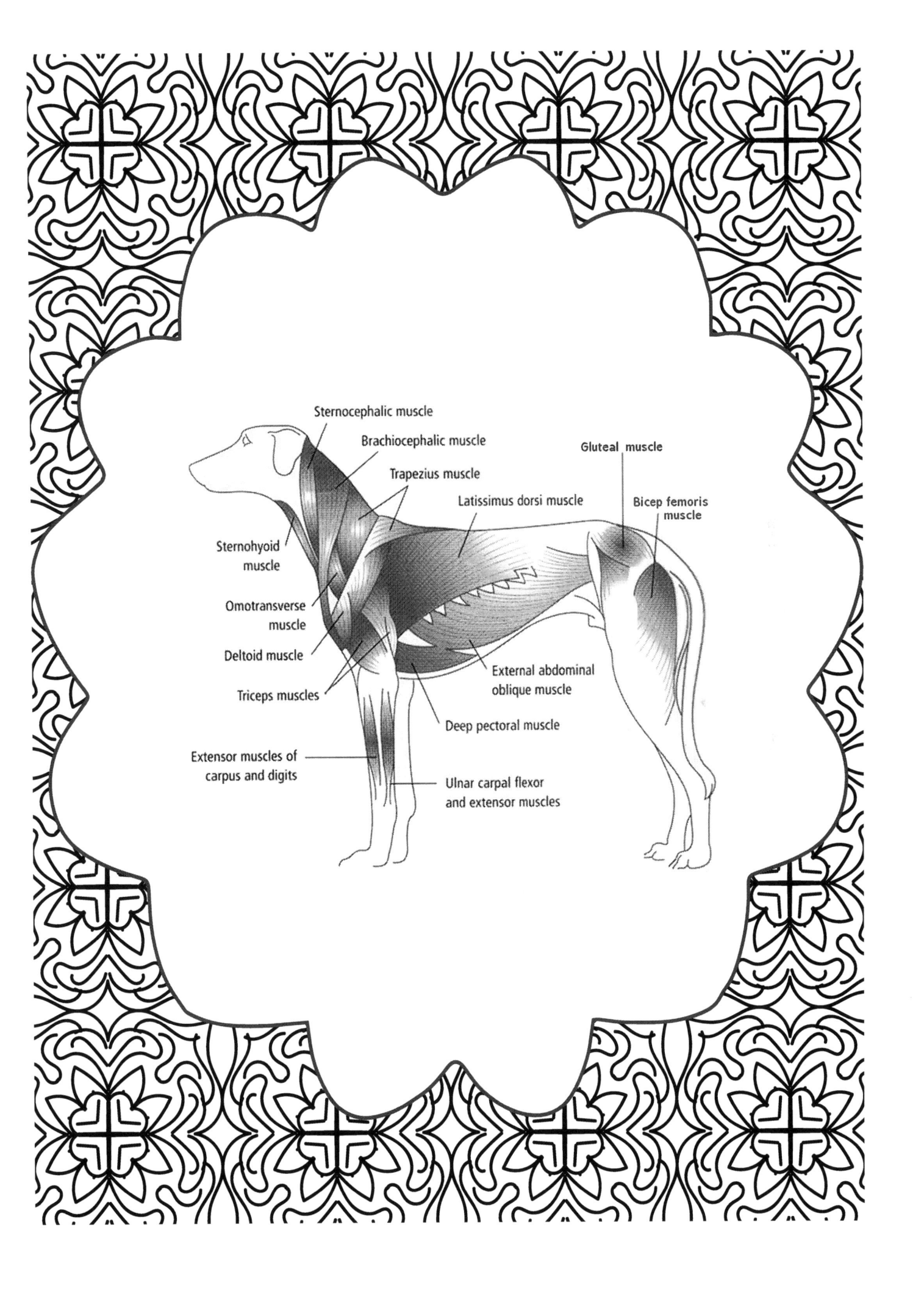

- Sternocephalic muscle
- Brachiocephalic muscle
- Trapezius muscle
- Latissimus dorsi muscle
- Gluteal muscle
- Bicep femoris muscle
- Sternohyoid muscle
- Omotransverse muscle
- Deltoid muscle
- Triceps muscles
- External abdominal oblique muscle
- Deep pectoral muscle
- Extensor muscles of carpus and digits
- Ulnar carpal flexor and extensor muscles

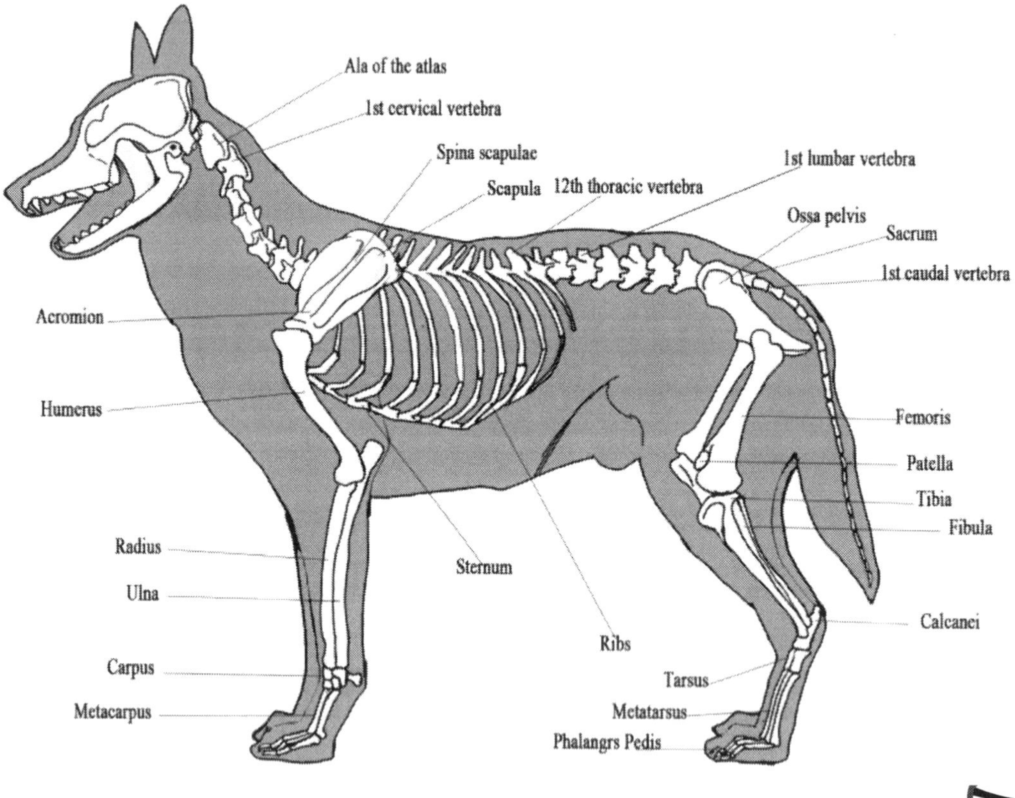
Ala of the atlas
1st cervical vertebra
Spina scapulae
Scapula
12th thoracic vertebra
1st lumbar vertebra
Ossa pelvis
Sacrum
1st caudal vertebra
Acromion
Humerus
Femoris
Patella
Tibia
Fibula
Radius
Sternum
Ulna
Calcanei
Ribs
Carpus
Tarsus
Metacarpus
Metatarsus
Phalangrs Pedis

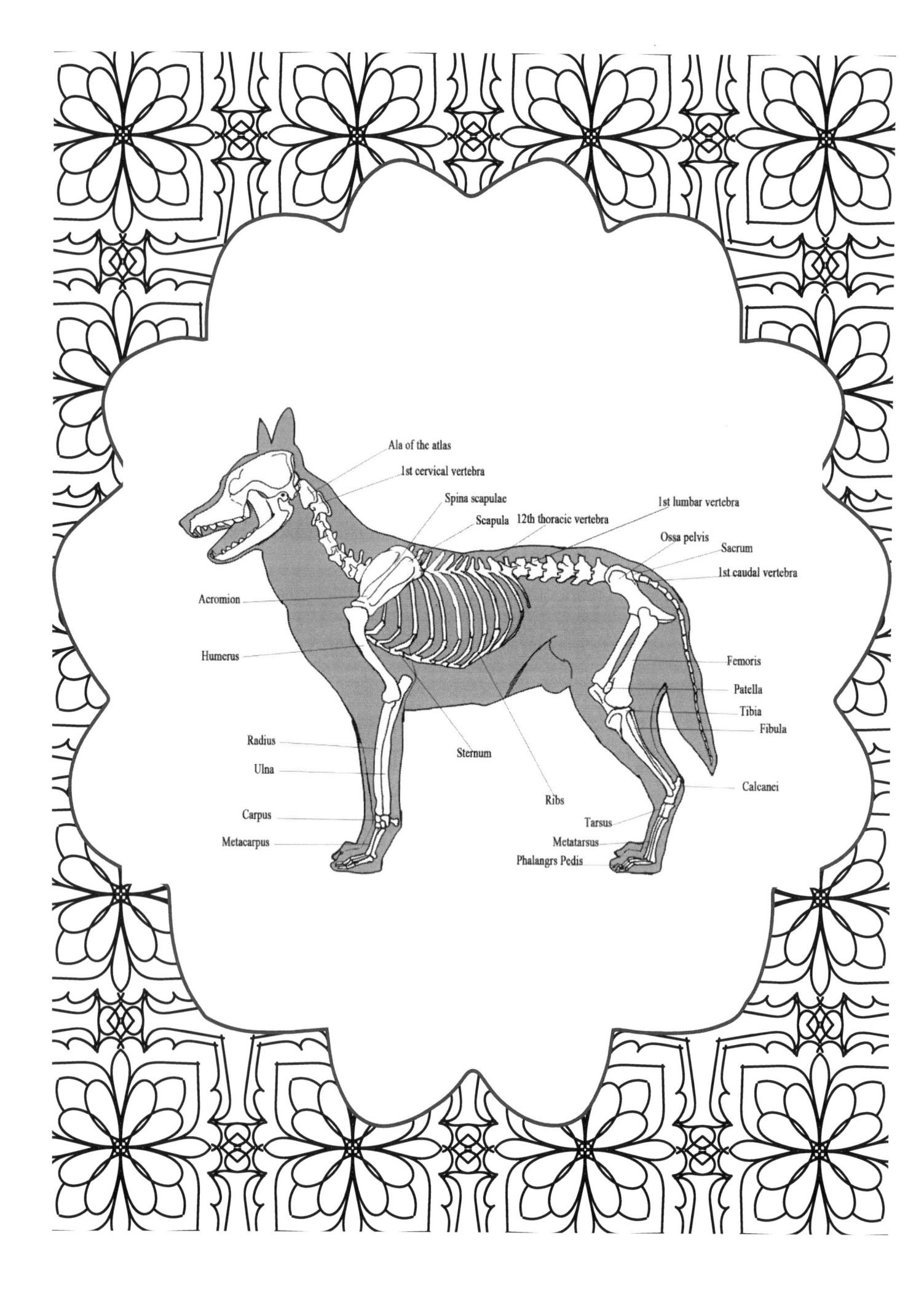

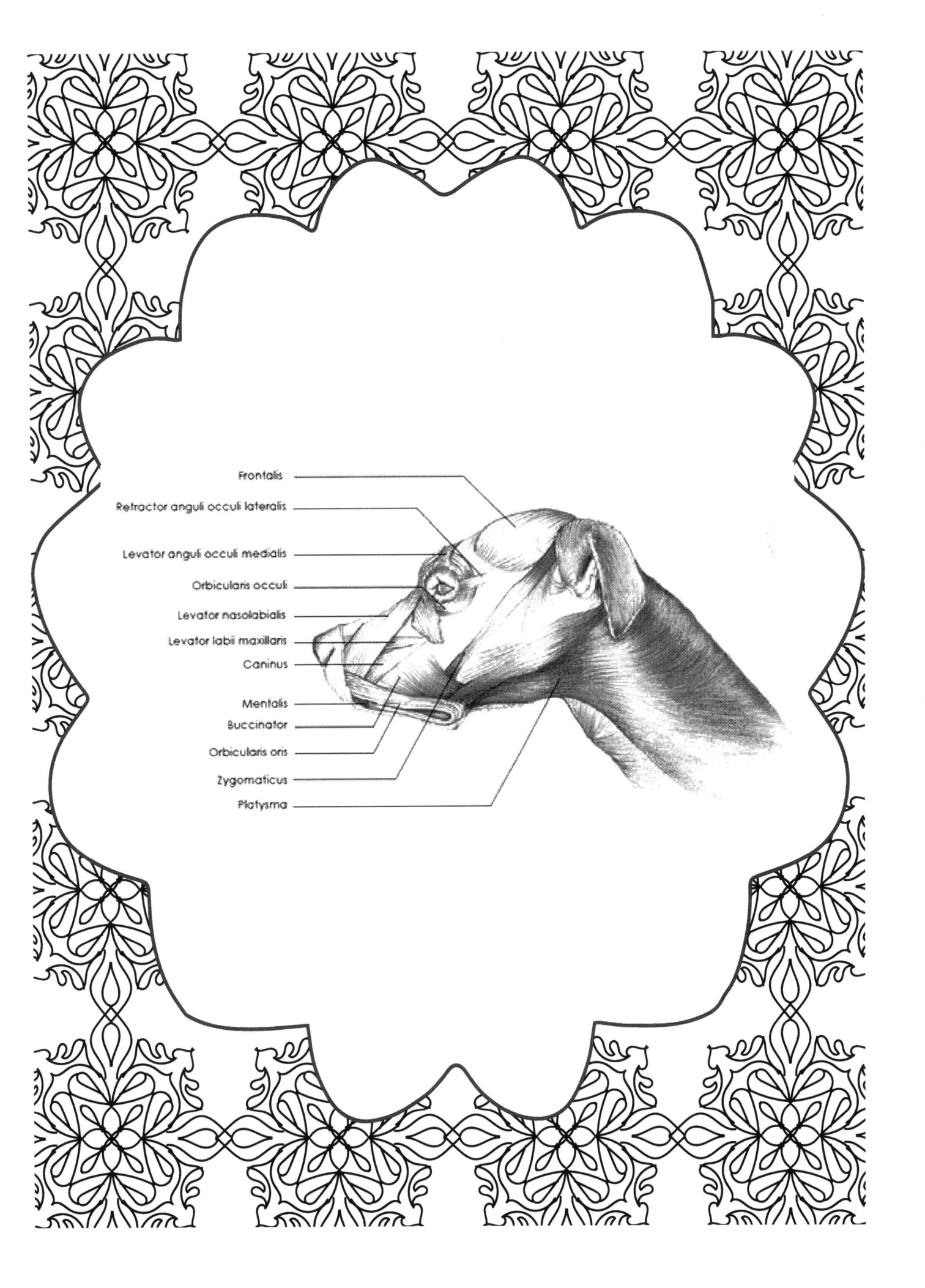

- Frontalis
- Retractor anguli occuli lateralis
- Levator anguli occuli medialis
- Orbicularis occuli
- Levator nasolabialis
- Levator labii maxillaris
- Caninus
- Mentalis
- Buccinator
- Orbicularis oris
- Zygomaticus
- Platysma

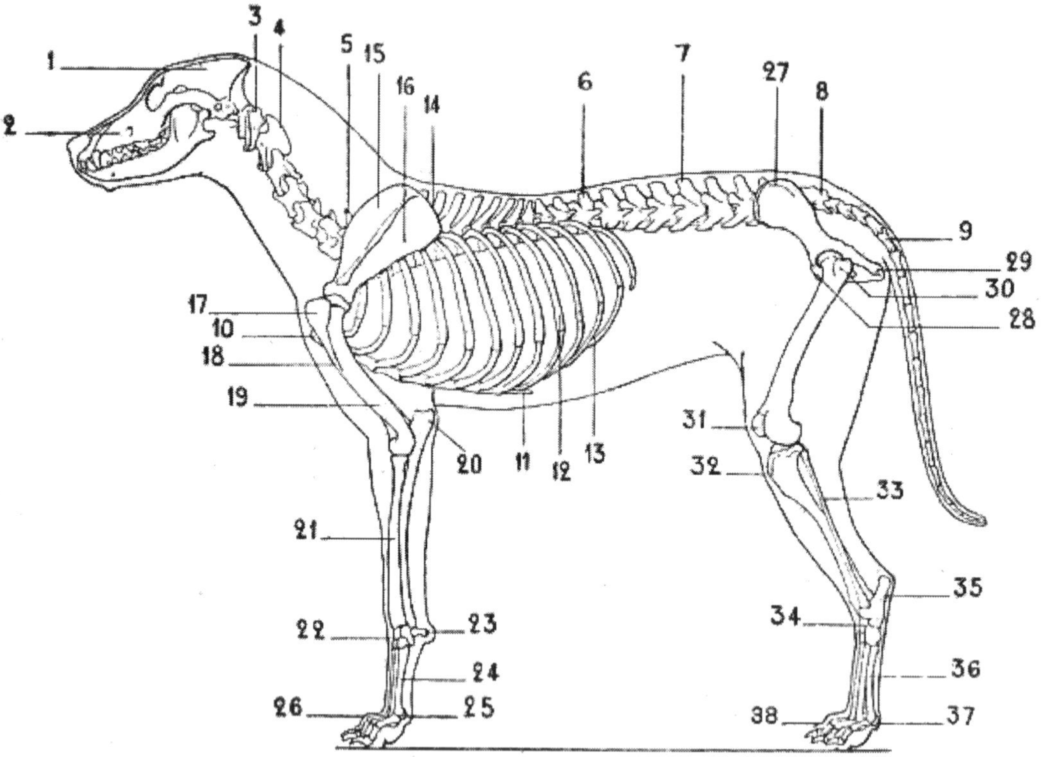
1
2
3
4
5
6
7
8
9
10
11
12
13
14
15
16
17
18
19
20
21
22
23
24
25
26
27
28
29
30
31
32
33
34
35
36
37
38

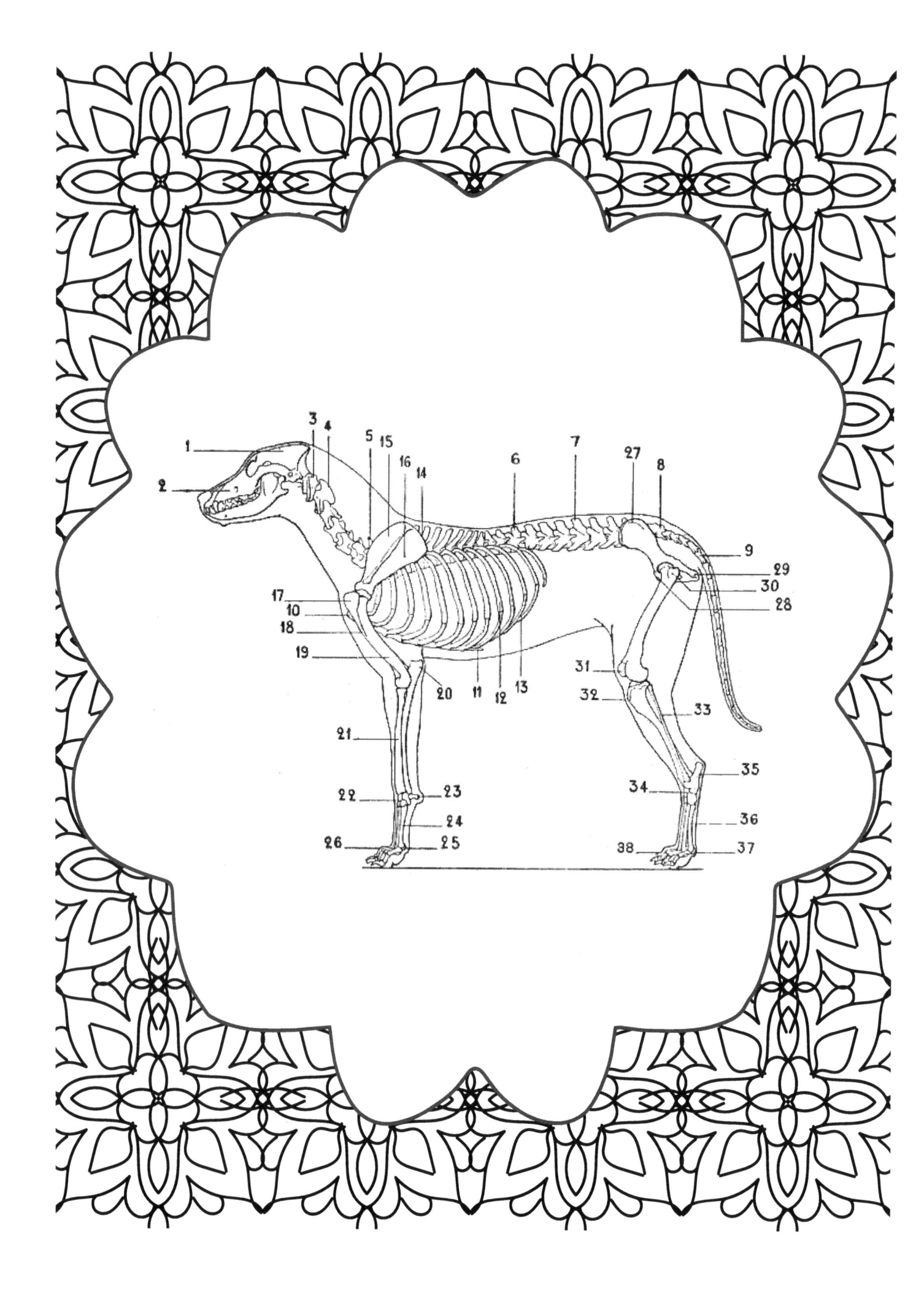

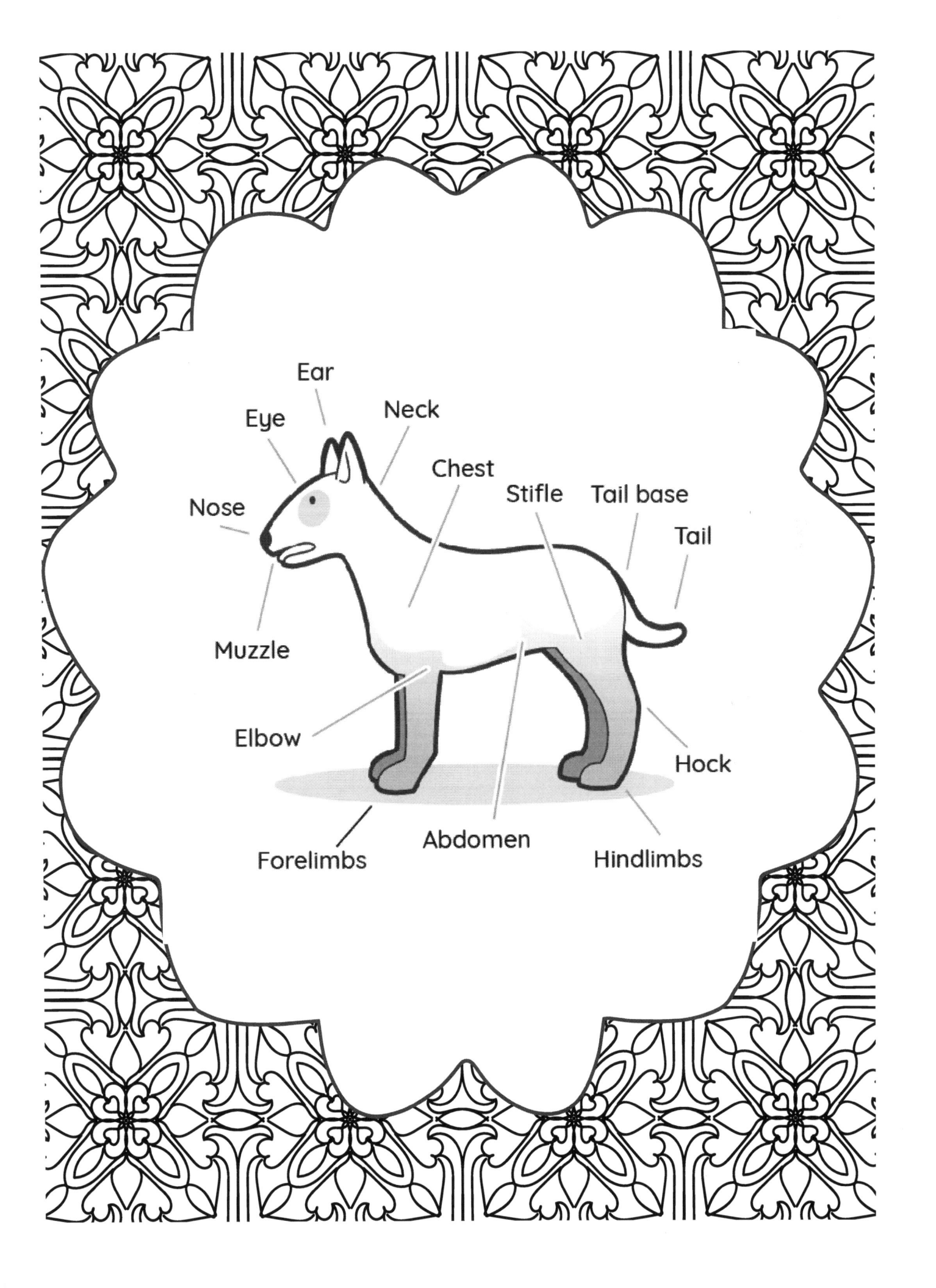

- Ear
- Eye
- Neck
- Nose
- Chest
- Stifle
- Tail base
- Tail
- Muzzle
- Elbow
- Hock
- Forelimbs
- Abdomen
- Hindlimbs

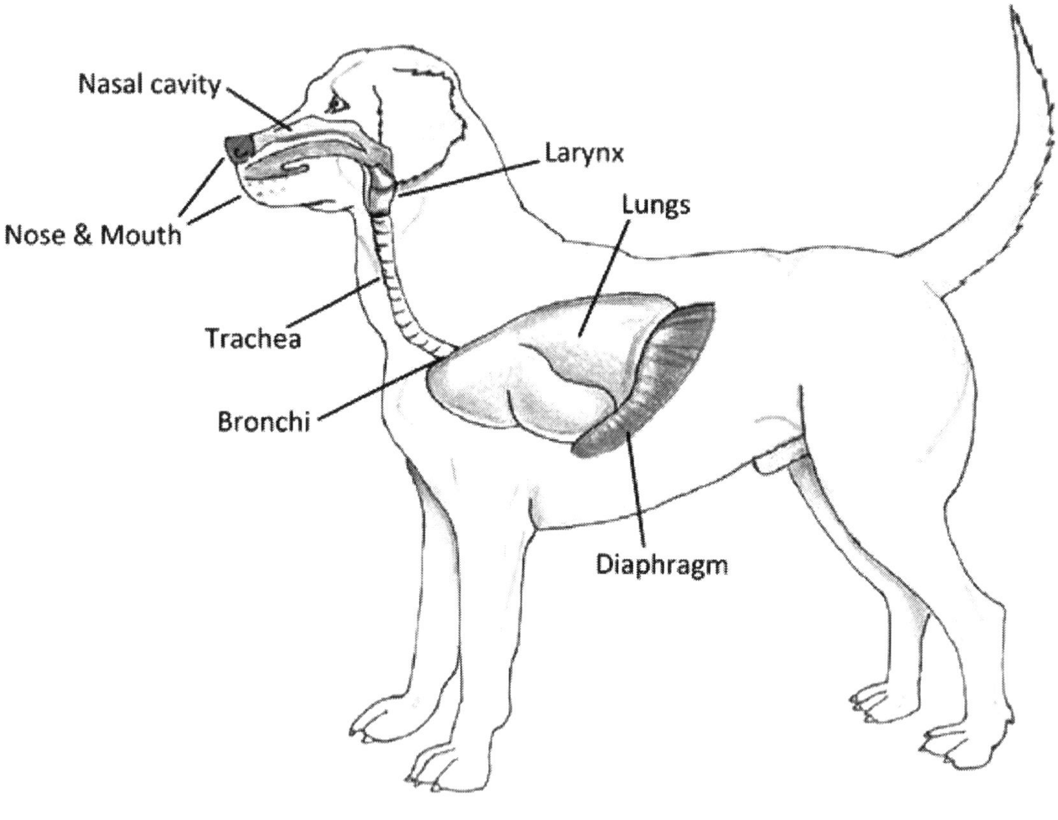
Nasal cavity
Larynx
Lungs
Nose & Mouth
Trachea
Bronchi
Diaphragm

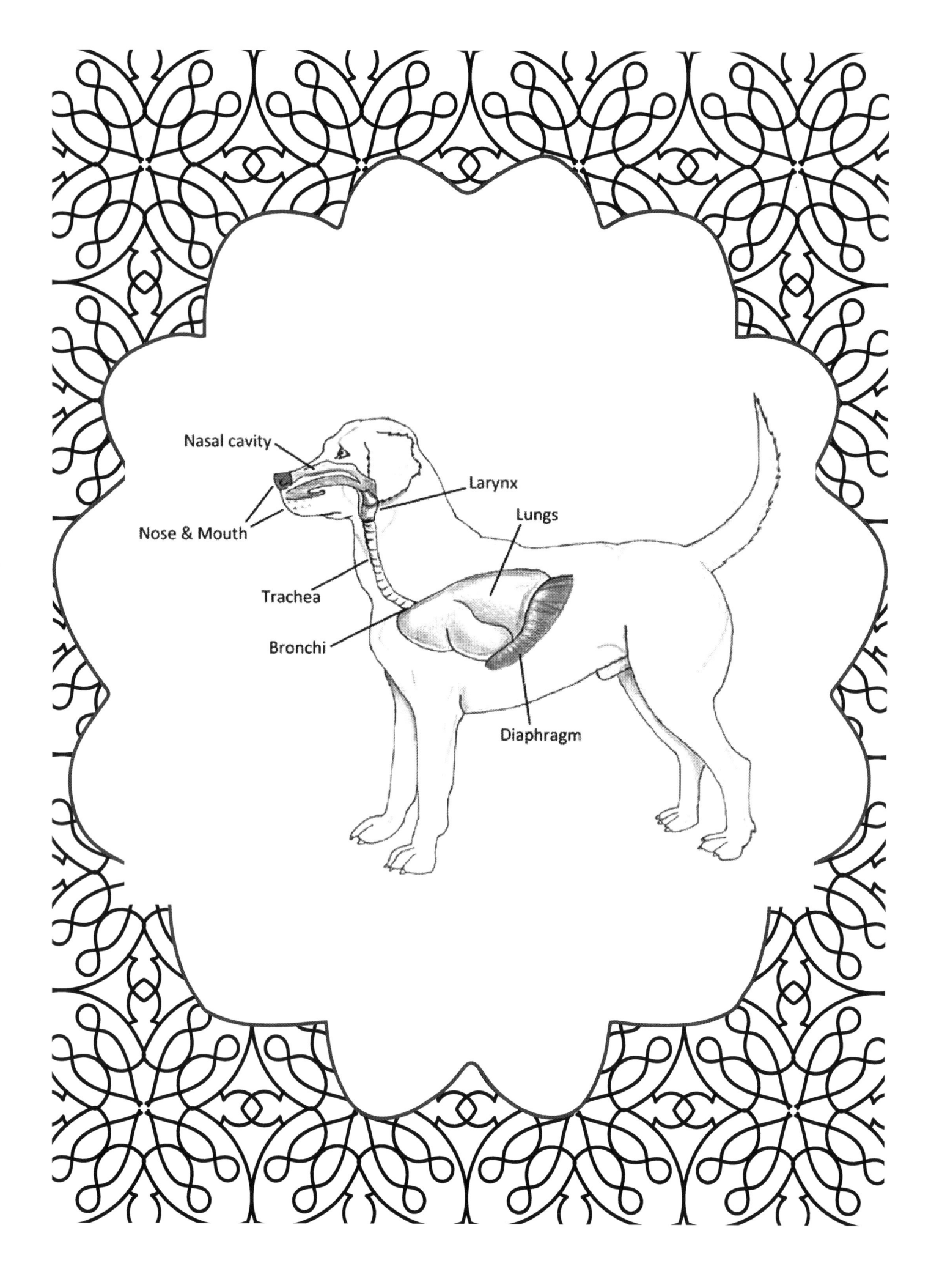

hock — stifle — knee

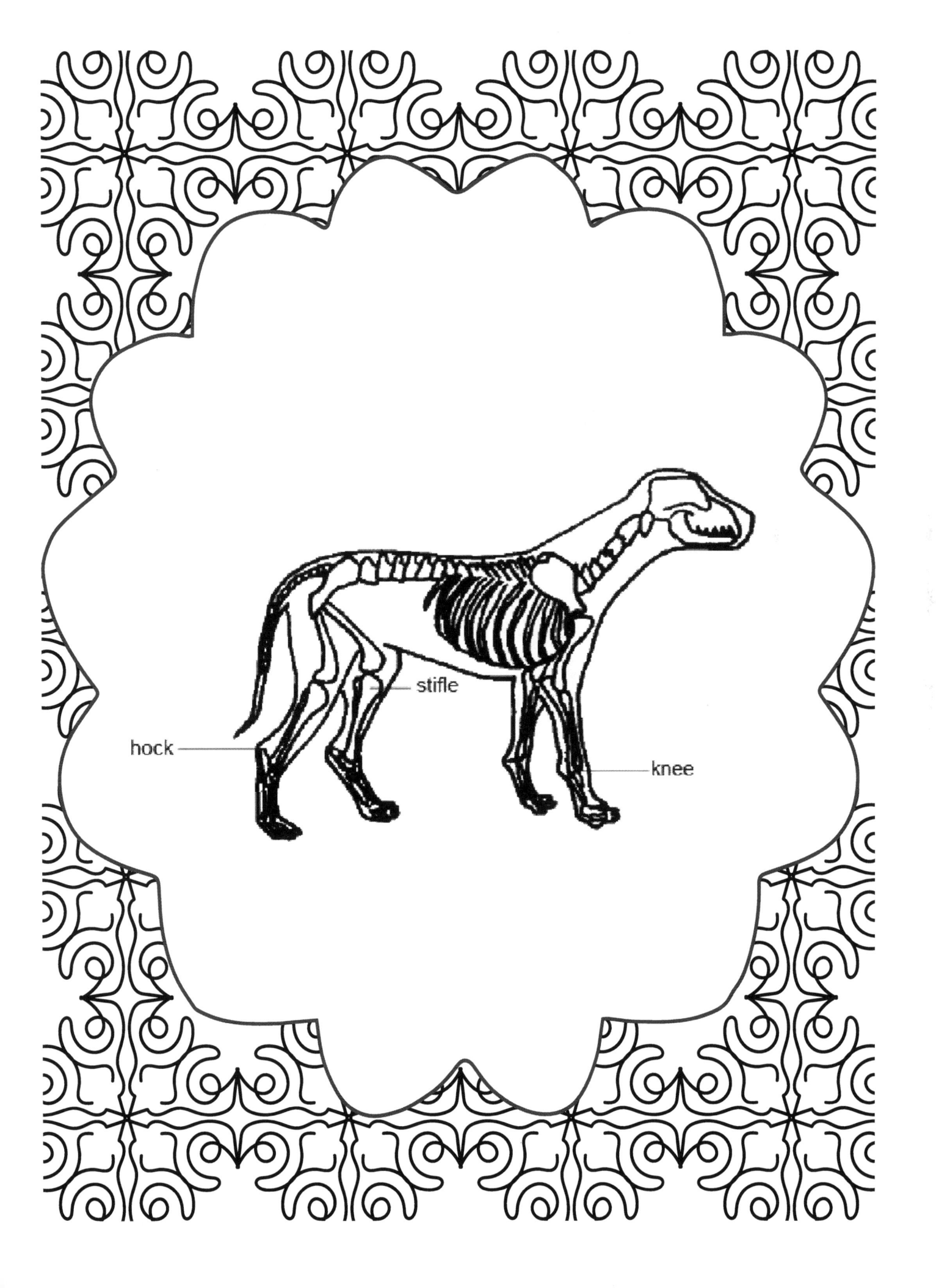

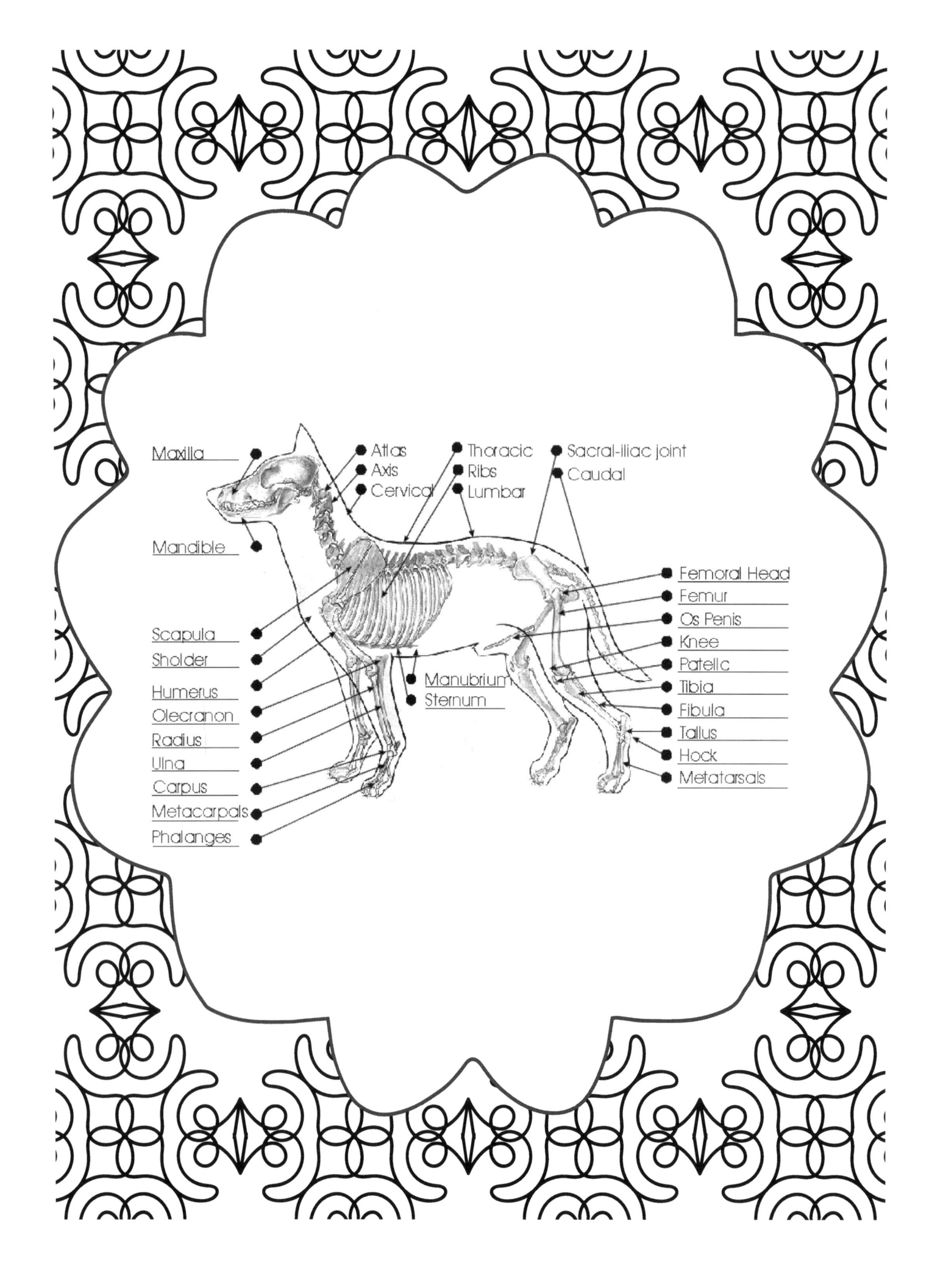

Maxilla	Atlas	Thoracic	Sacral-iliac joint
	Axis	Ribs	Caudal
	Cervical	Lumbar	

Mandible

Scapula
Sholder
Humerus
Olecranon
Radius
Ulna
Carpus
Metacarpals
Phalanges

Manubrium
Sternum

Femoral Head
Femur
Os Penis
Knee
Patella
Tibia
Fibula
Tallus
Hock
Metatarsals

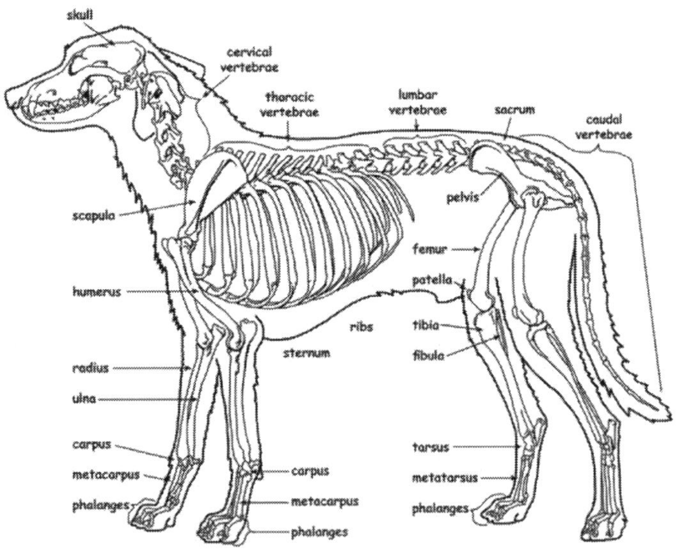
skull
cervical vertebrae
thoracic vertebrae
lumbar vertebrae
sacrum
caudal vertebrae
scapula
pelvis
femur
humerus
patella
ribs
tibia
radius
sternum
fibula
ulna
carpus
tarsus
metacarpus
carpus
metatarsus
phalanges
metacarpus
phalanges
phalanges

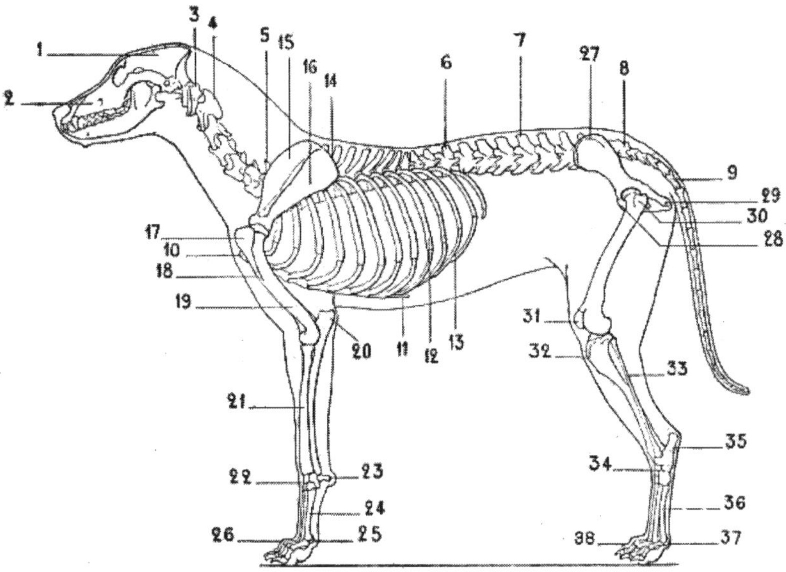
3
4
5
15
1
16
14
6
7
27
8
2
9
29
30
17
28
10
18
19
31
20
11
12
13
32
33
21
35
34
22
23
36
24
26
25
38
37

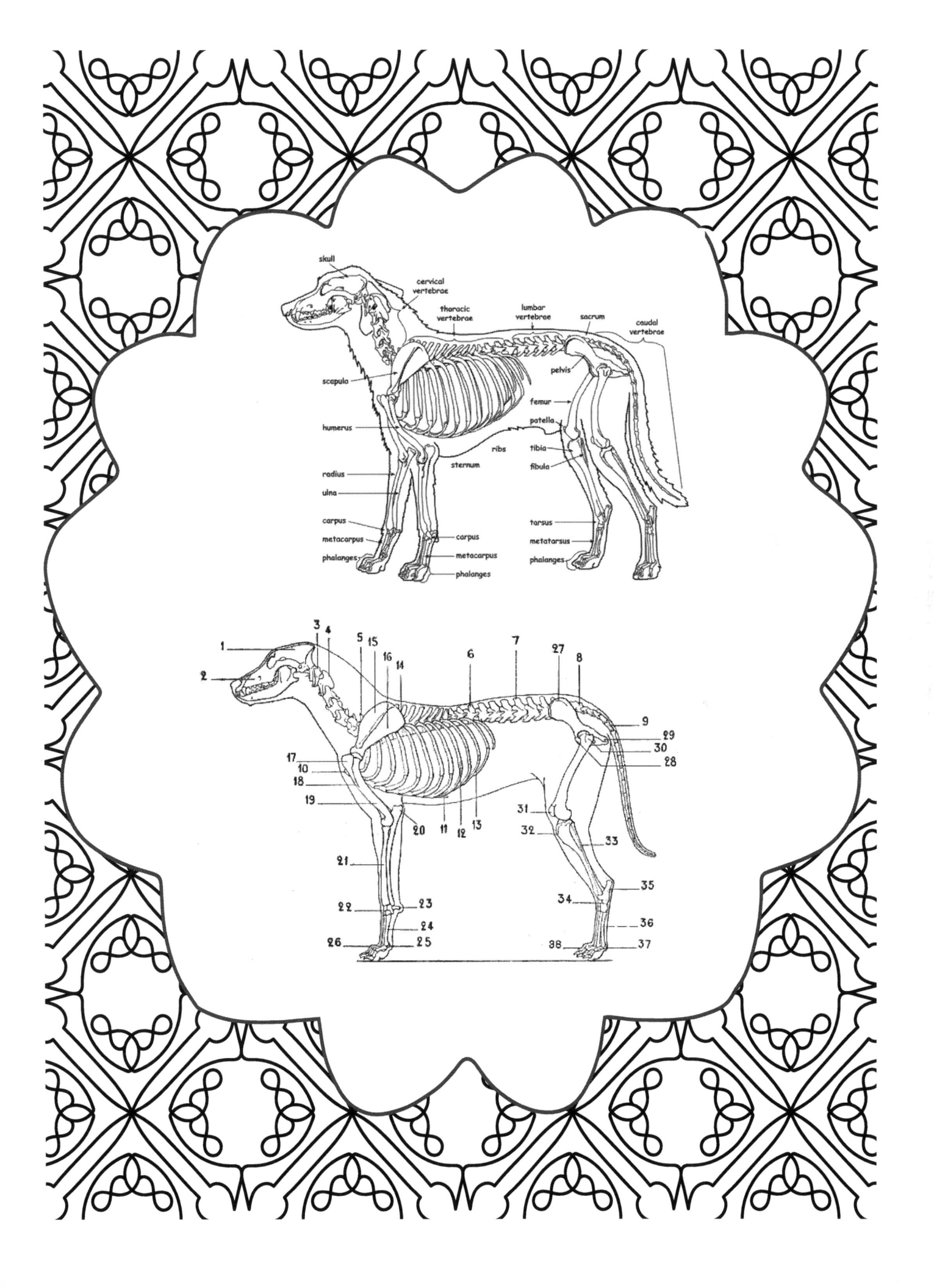

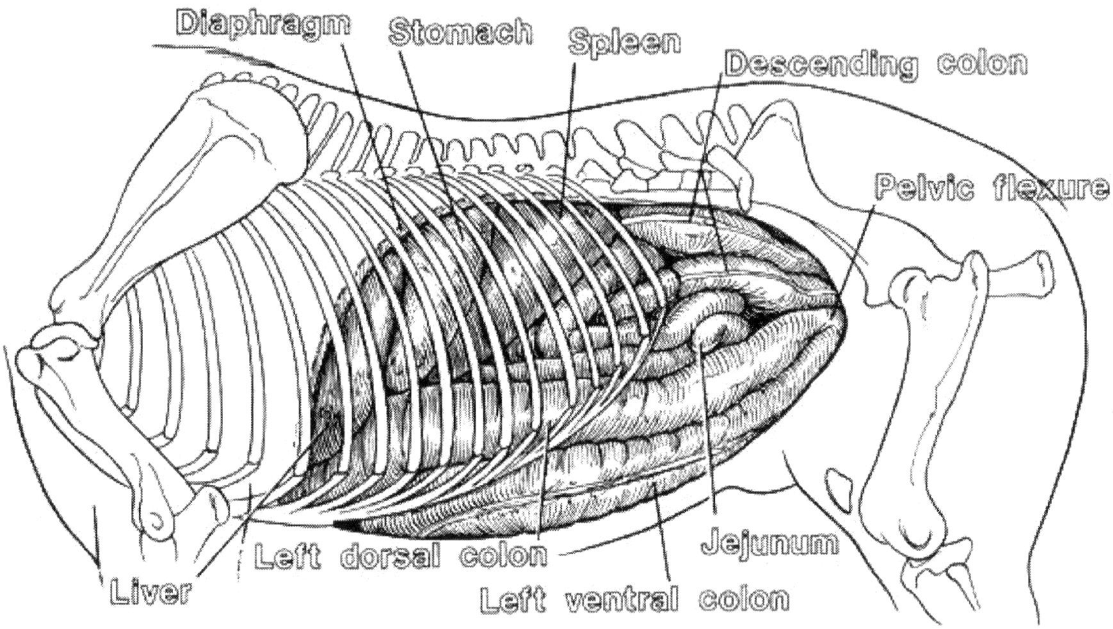
Diaphragm
Stomach
Spleen
Descending colon
Pelvic flexure
Jejunum
Left dorsal colon
Liver
Left ventral colon

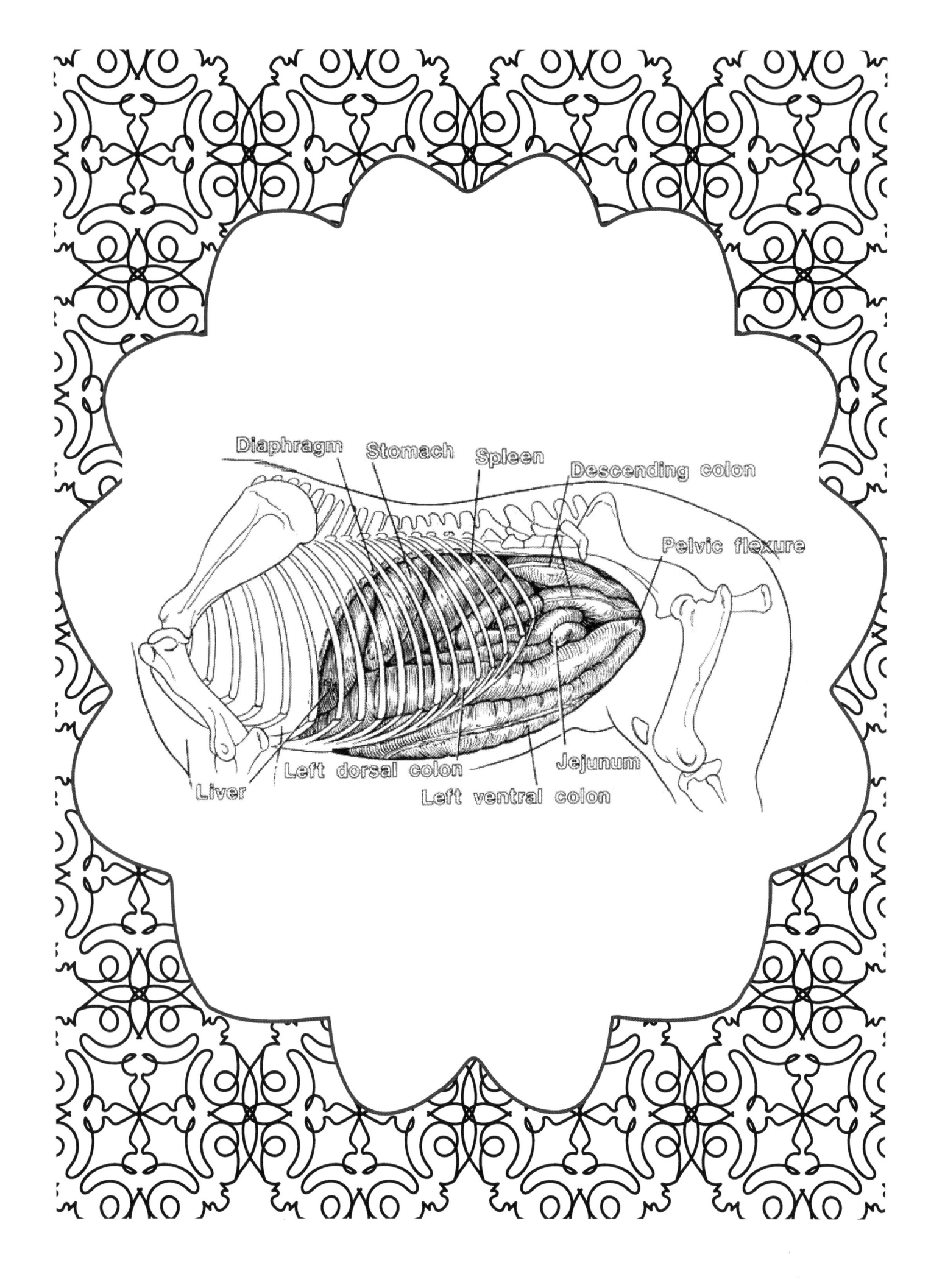

LENGTH

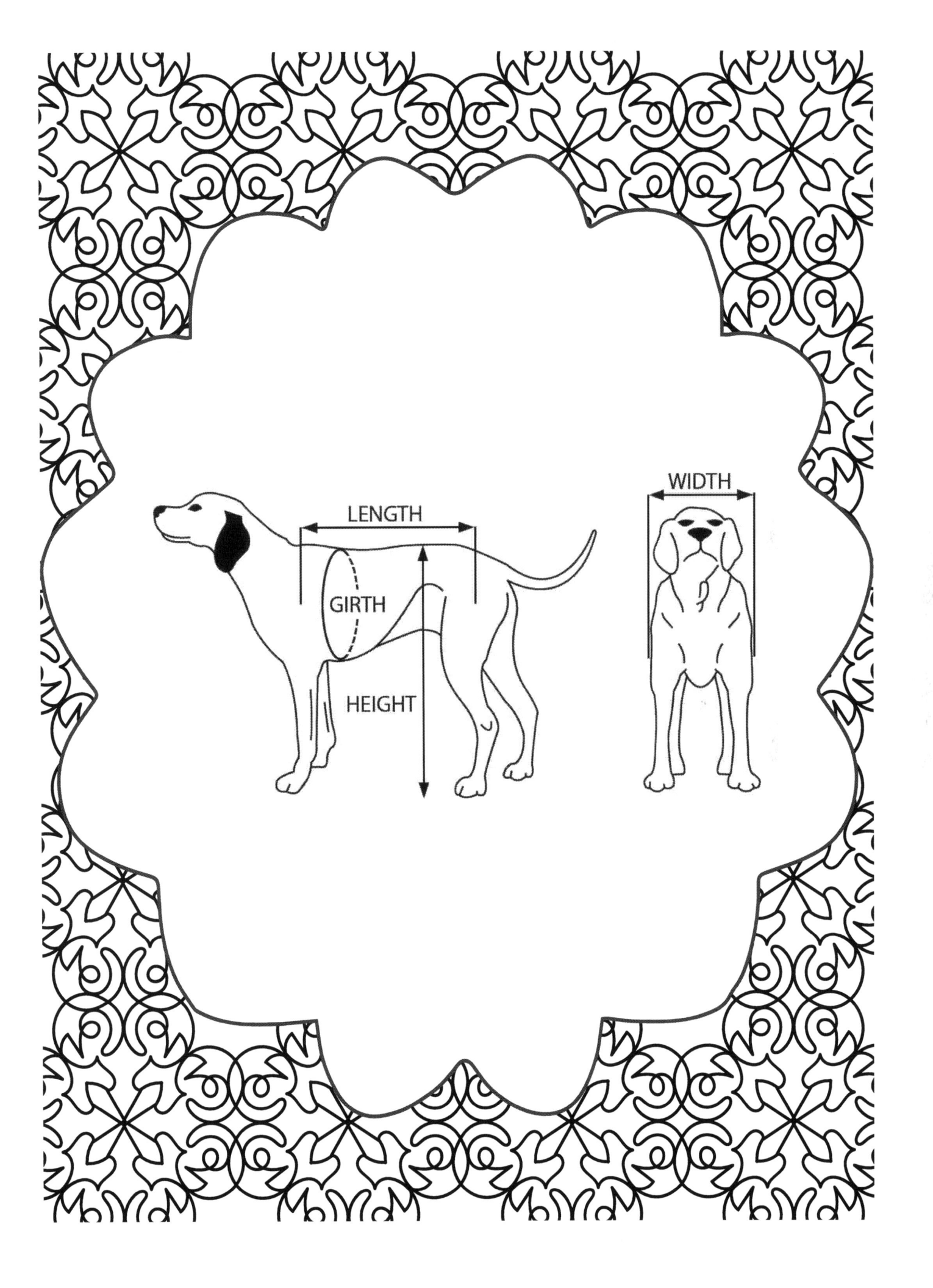

GIRTH

HEIGHT

WIDTH

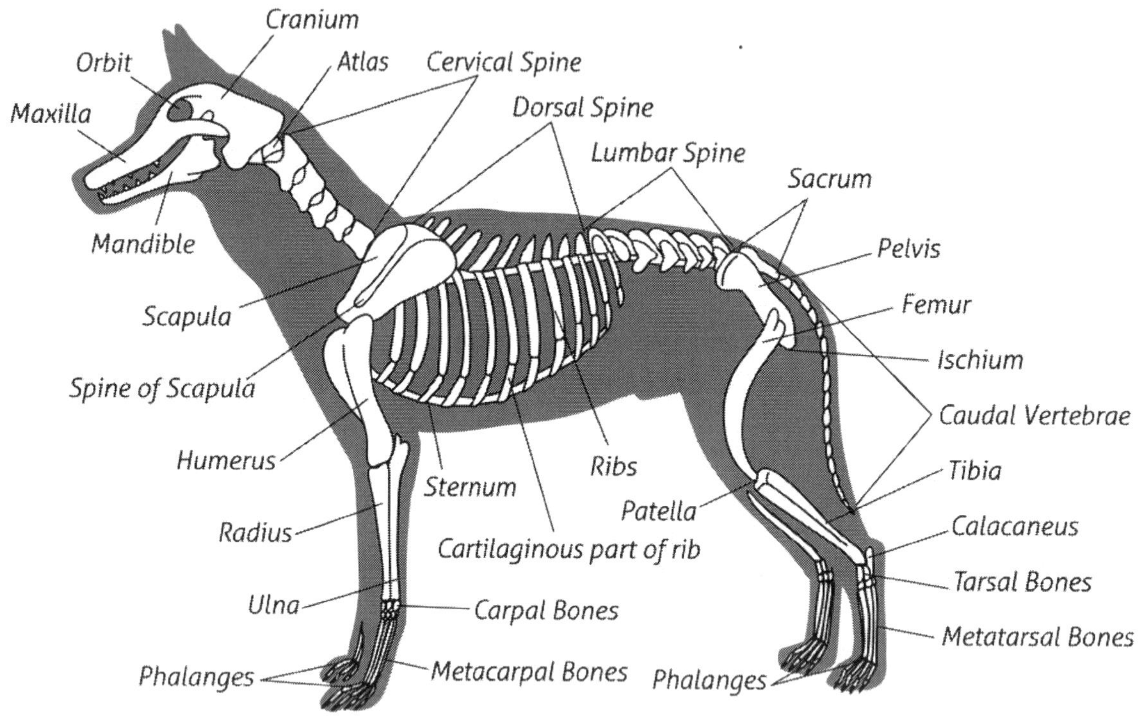
Cranium
Orbit
Atlas
Cervical Spine
Maxilla
Dorsal Spine
Lumbar Spine
Sacrum
Mandible
Pelvis
Scapula
Femur
Spine of Scapula
Ischium
Caudal Vertebrae
Humerus
Ribs
Tibia
Sternum
Patella
Radius
Calacaneus
Cartilaginous part of rib
Tarsal Bones
Ulna
Carpal Bones
Metatarsal Bones
Phalanges
Metacarpal Bones
Phalanges

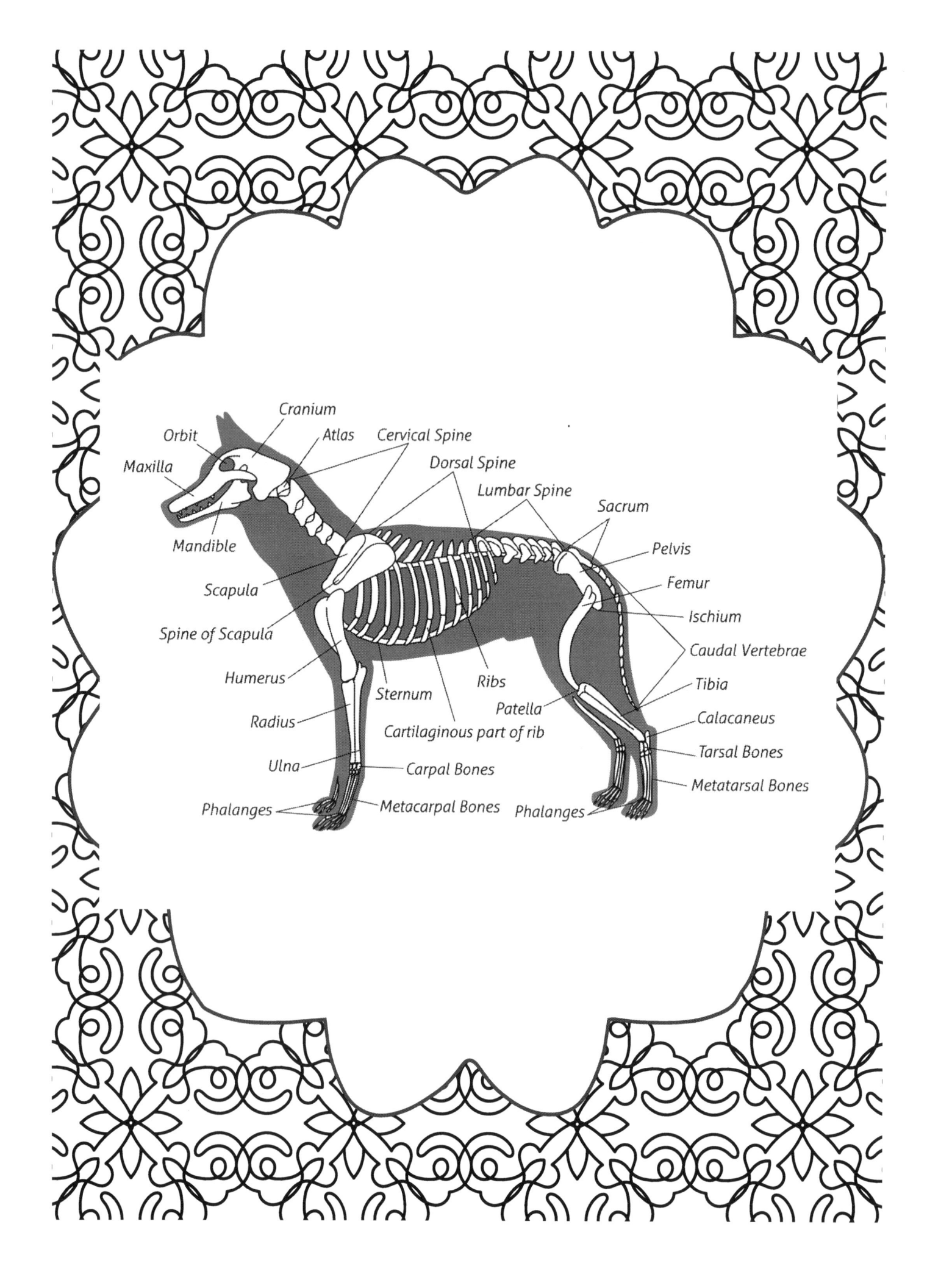

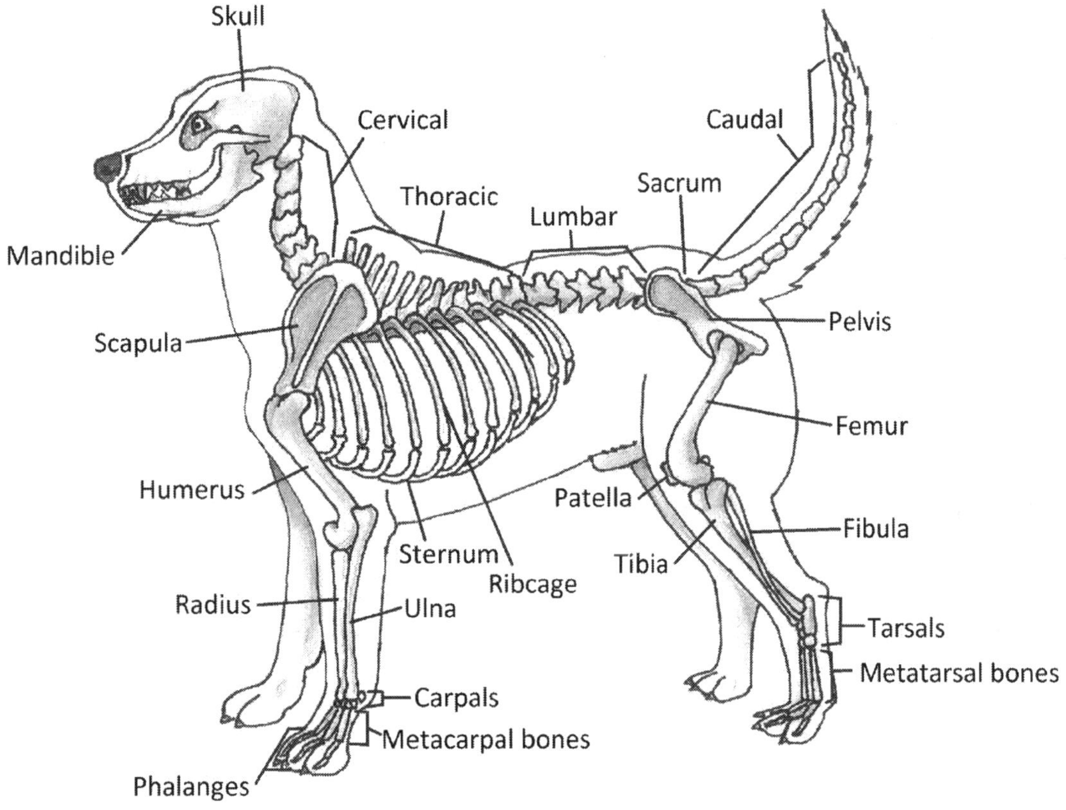
Skull
Cervical
Caudal
Thoracic
Sacrum
Lumbar
Mandible
Pelvis
Scapula
Femur
Humerus
Patella
Fibula
Sternum
Tibia
Ribcage
Radius
Ulna
Tarsals
Metatarsal bones
Carpals
Metacarpal bones
Phalanges

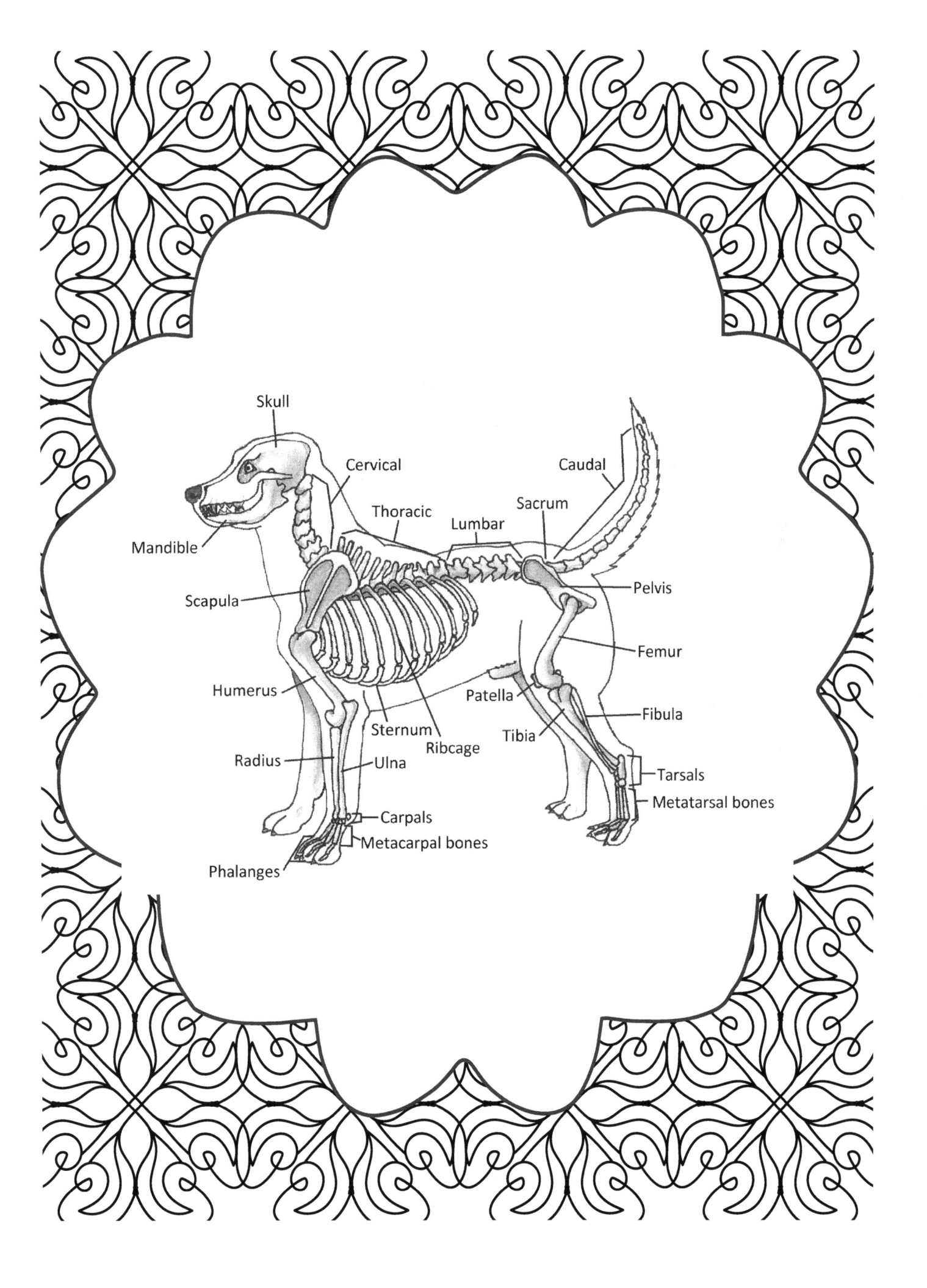

ANATOMY OF A DOG

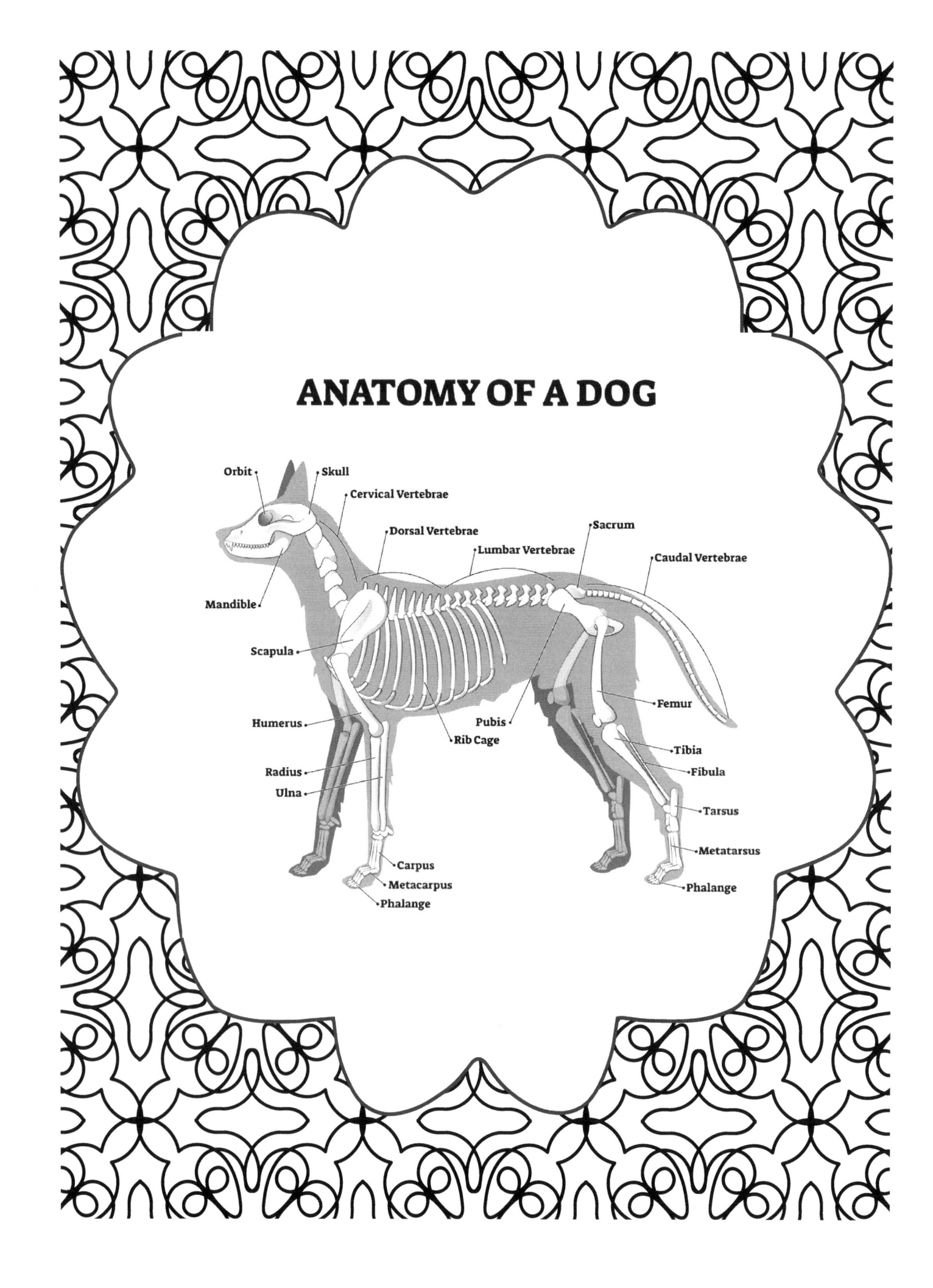

- Orbit
- Skull
- Cervical Vertebrae
- Dorsal Vertebrae
- Sacrum
- Lumbar Vertebrae
- Caudal Vertebrae
- Mandible
- Scapula
- Humerus
- Pubis
- Rib Cage
- Femur
- Tibia
- Fibula
- Radius
- Ulna
- Tarsus
- Metatarsus
- Carpus
- Metacarpus
- Phalange
- Phalange

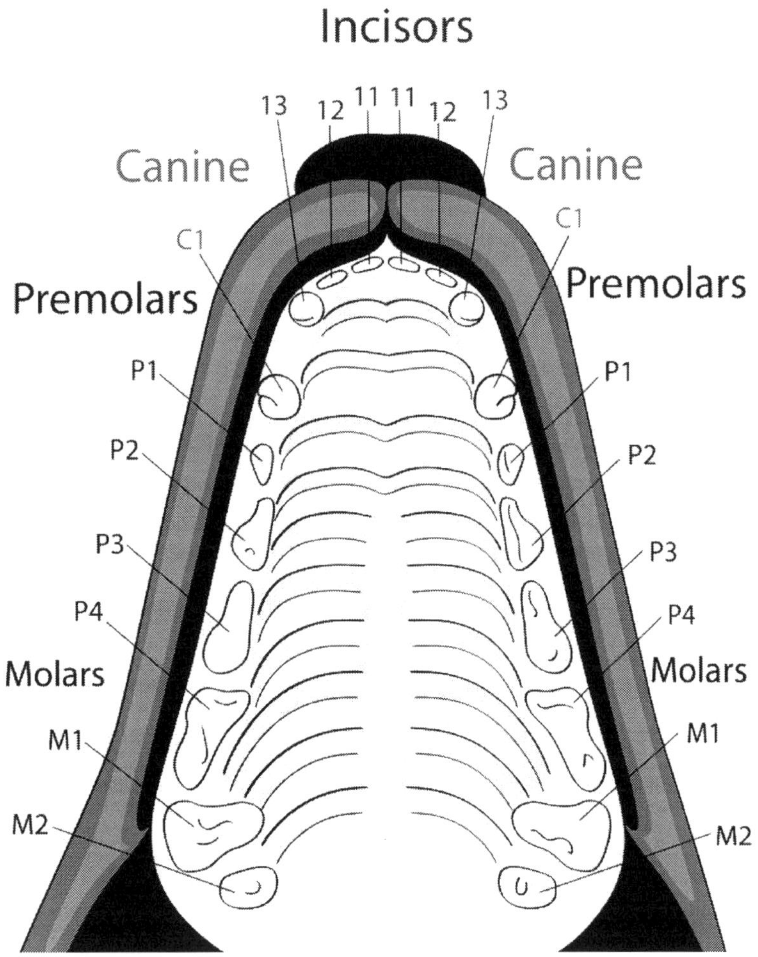
Incisors
13
12
11
11
12
13
Canine
Canine
C1
C1
Premolars
Premolars
P1
P1
P2
P2
P3
P3
P4
P4
Molars
Molars
M1
M1
M2
M2

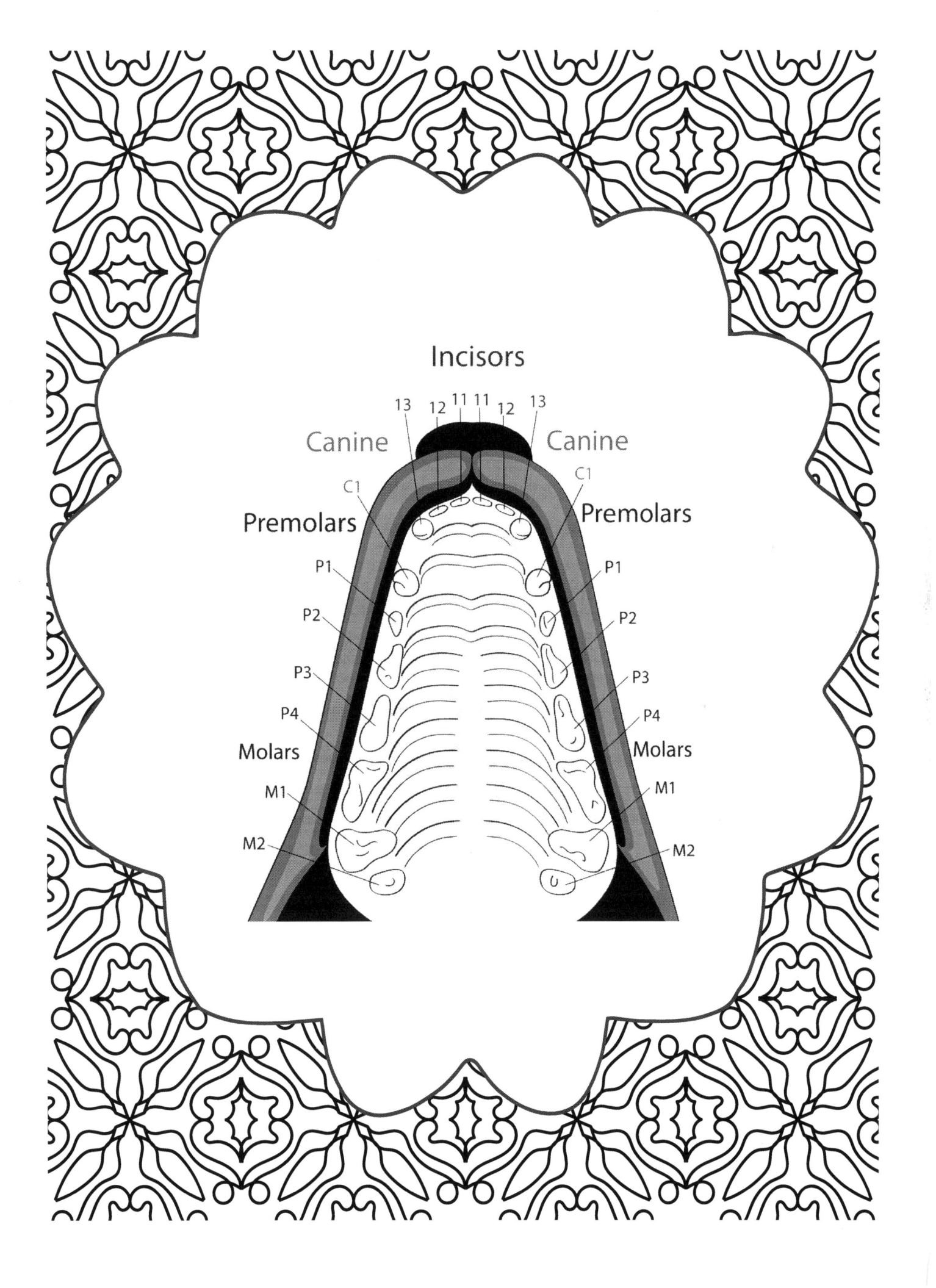

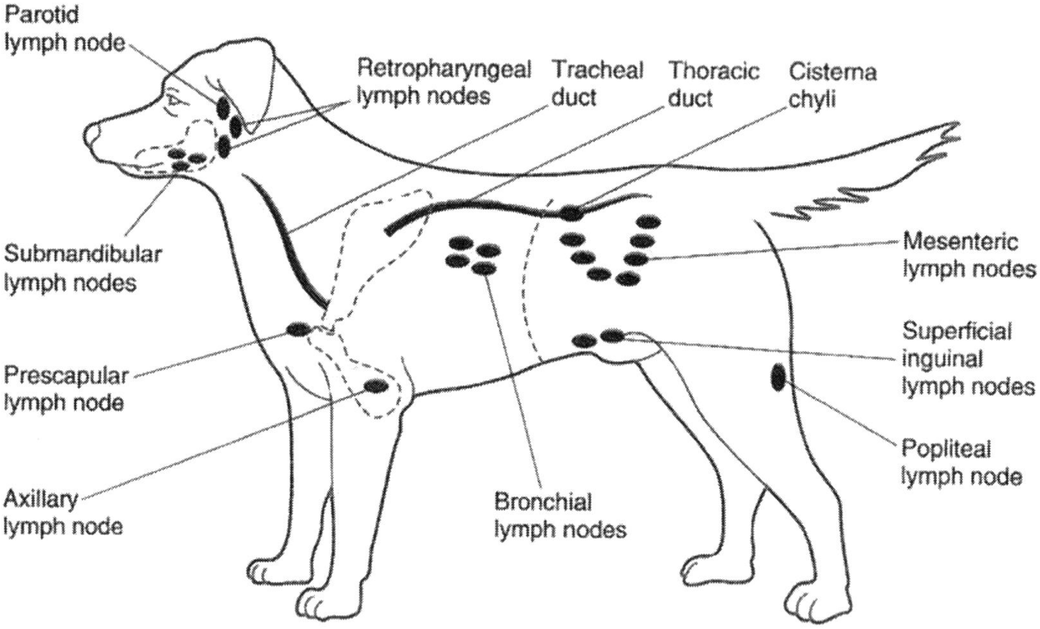

Parotid lymph node
Retropharyngeal lymph nodes
Tracheal duct
Thoracic duct
Cisterna chyli
Submandibular lymph nodes
Mesenteric lymph nodes
Superficial inguinal lymph nodes
Prescapular lymph node
Popliteal lymph node
Axillary lymph node
Bronchial lymph nodes

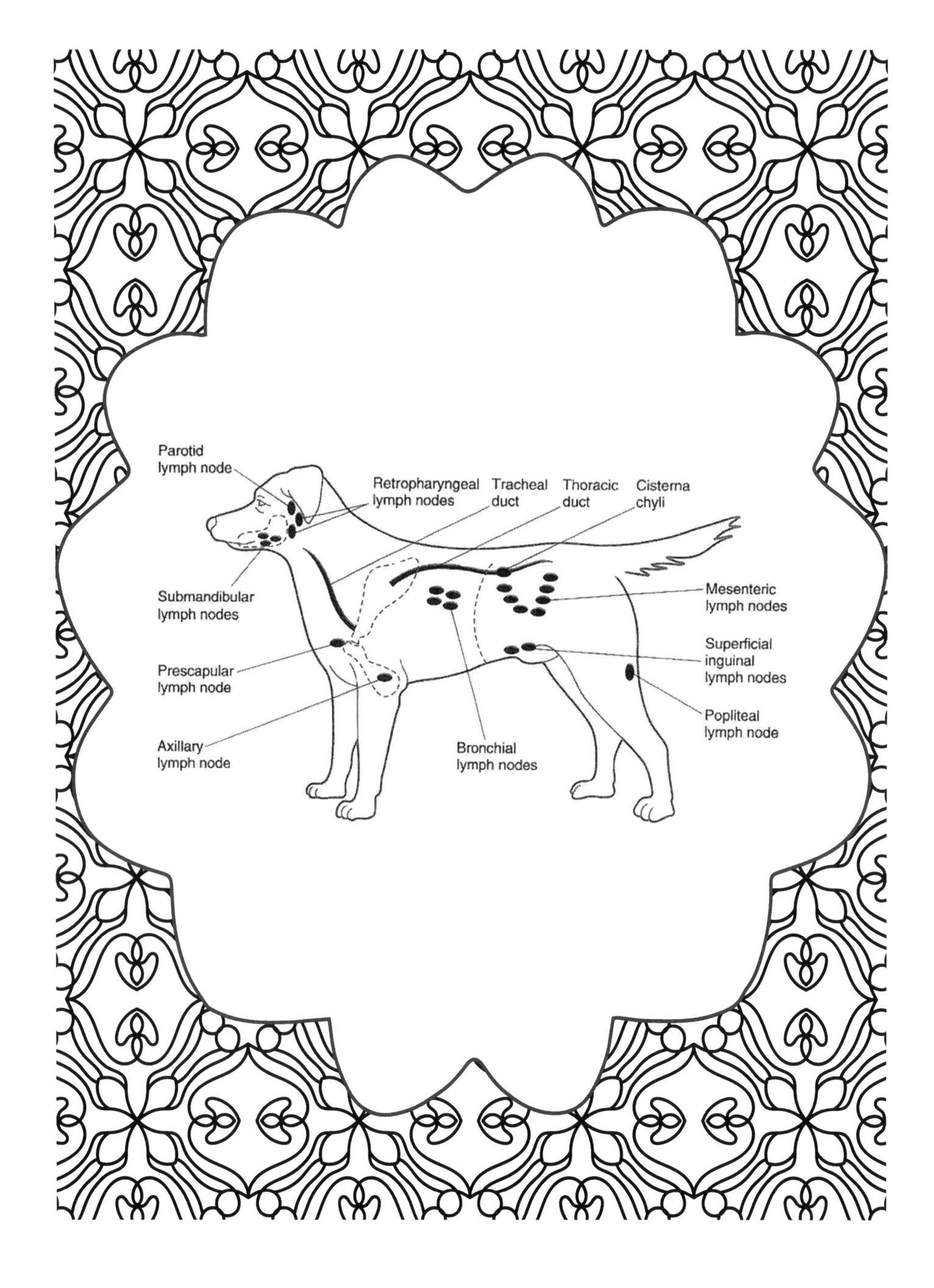

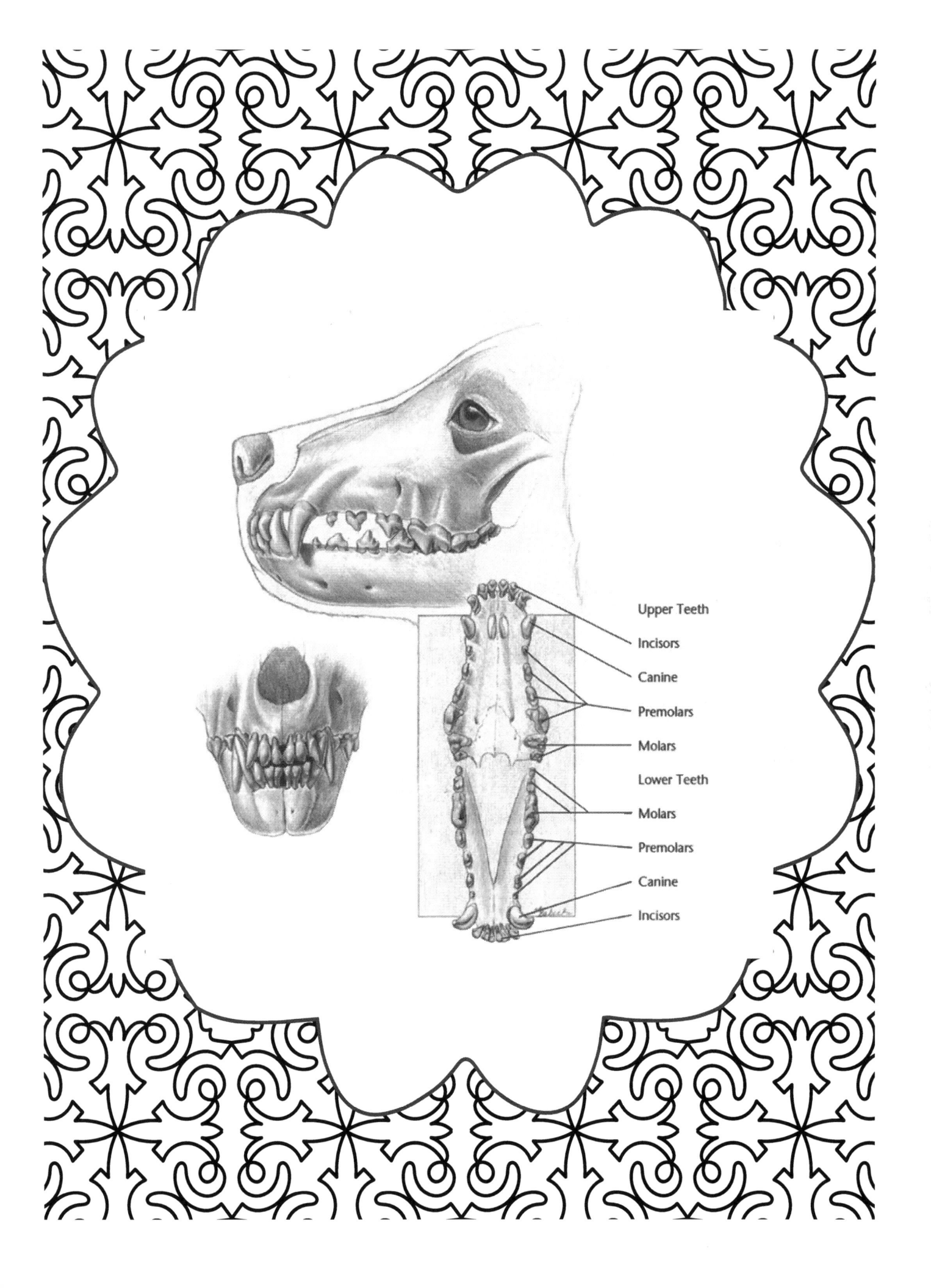

Upper Teeth
Incisors
Canine
Premolars
Molars
Lower Teeth
Molars
Premolars
Canine
Incisors

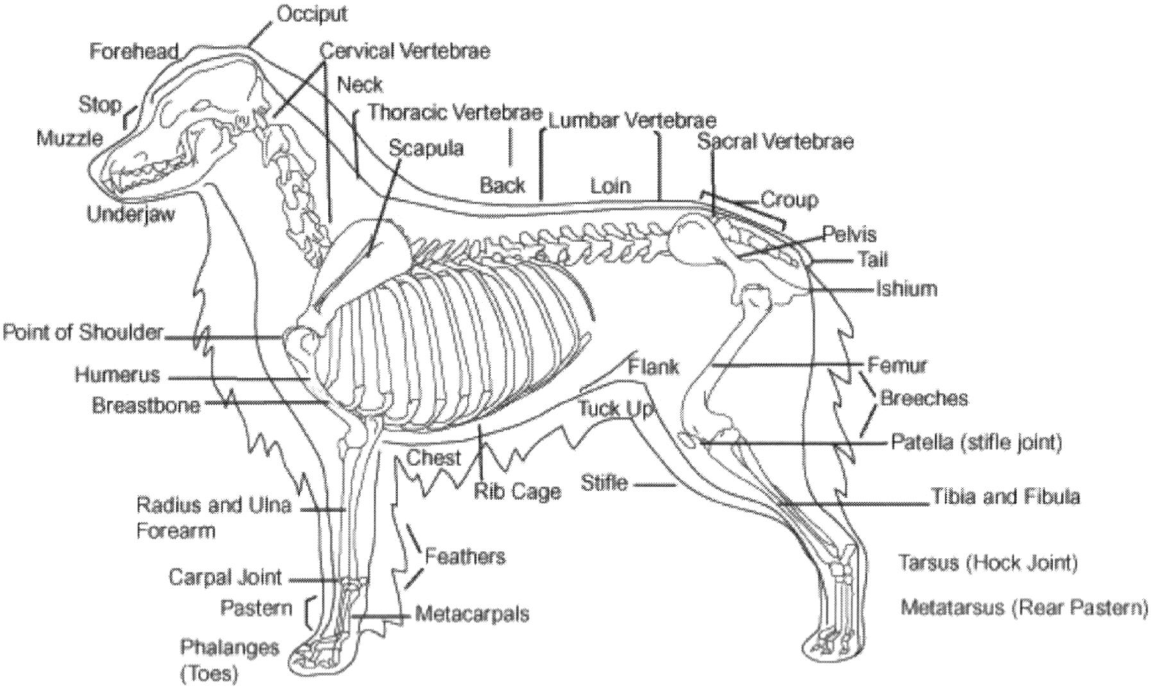
Occiput
Forehead
Cervical Vertebrae
Neck
Stop
Thoracic Vertebrae
Lumbar Vertebrae
Muzzle
Scapula
Sacral Vertebrae
Back
Loin
Croup
Underjaw
Pelvis
Tail
Ishium
Point of Shoulder
Flank
Femur
Humerus
Breeches
Breastbone
Tuck Up
Patella (stifle joint)
Chest
Stifle
Rib Cage
Tibia and Fibula
Radius and Ulna
Forearm
Feathers
Tarsus (Hock Joint)
Carpal Joint
Pastern
Metacarpals
Metatarsus (Rear Pastern)
Phalanges
(Toes)

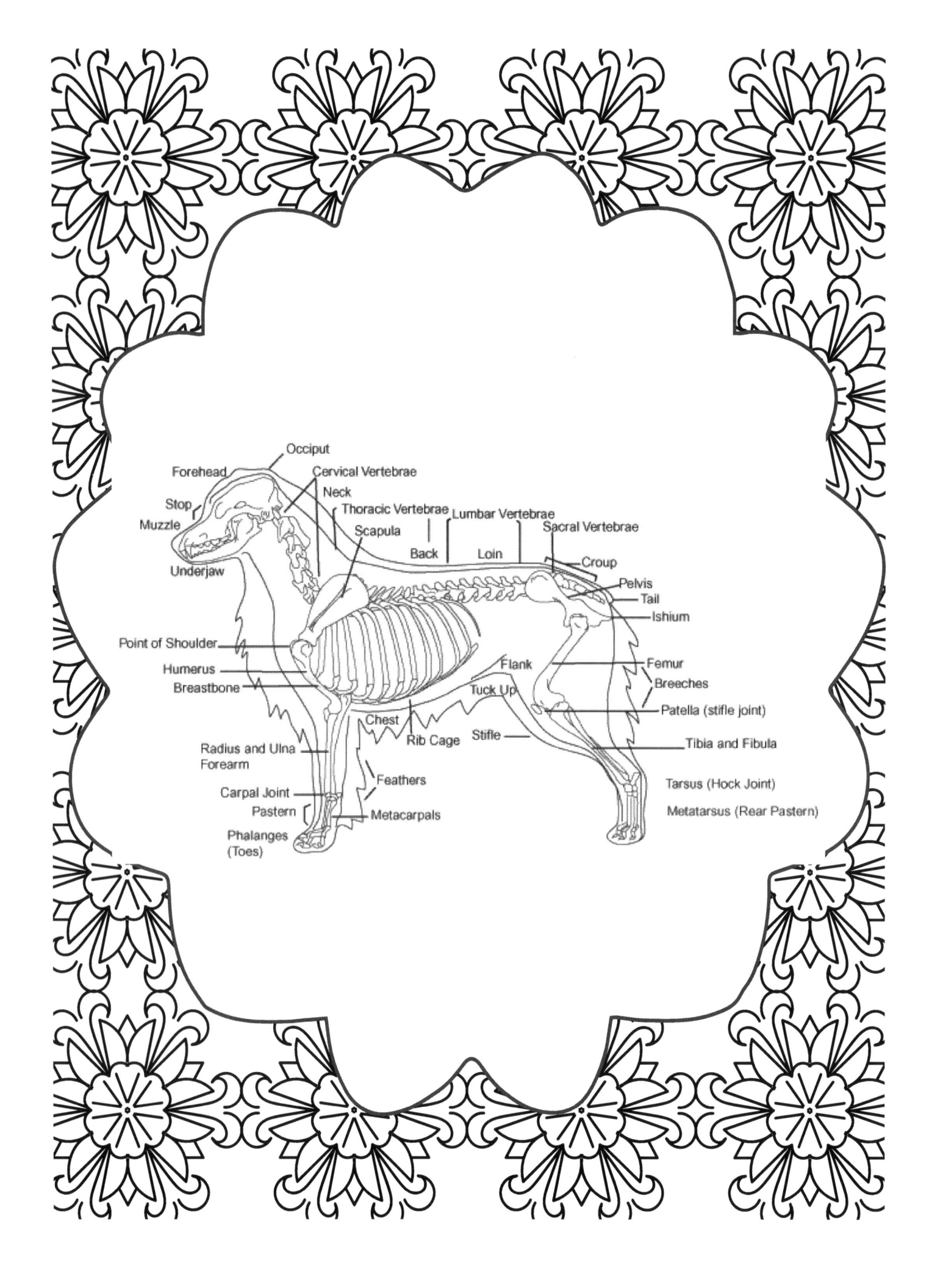

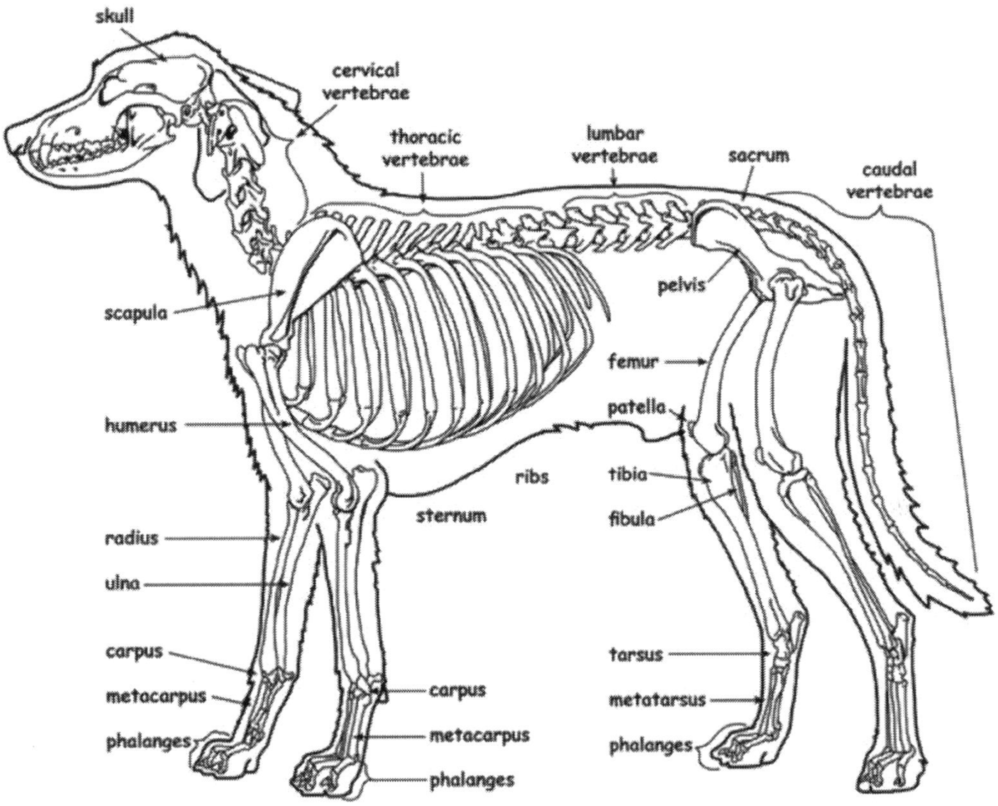
skull
cervical vertebrae
thoracic vertebrae
lumbar vertebrae
sacrum
caudal vertebrae
pelvis
scapula
femur
patella
humerus
ribs
tibia
fibula
sternum
radius
ulna
carpus
metacarpus
phalanges
carpus
metacarpus
phalanges
tarsus
metatarsus
phalanges

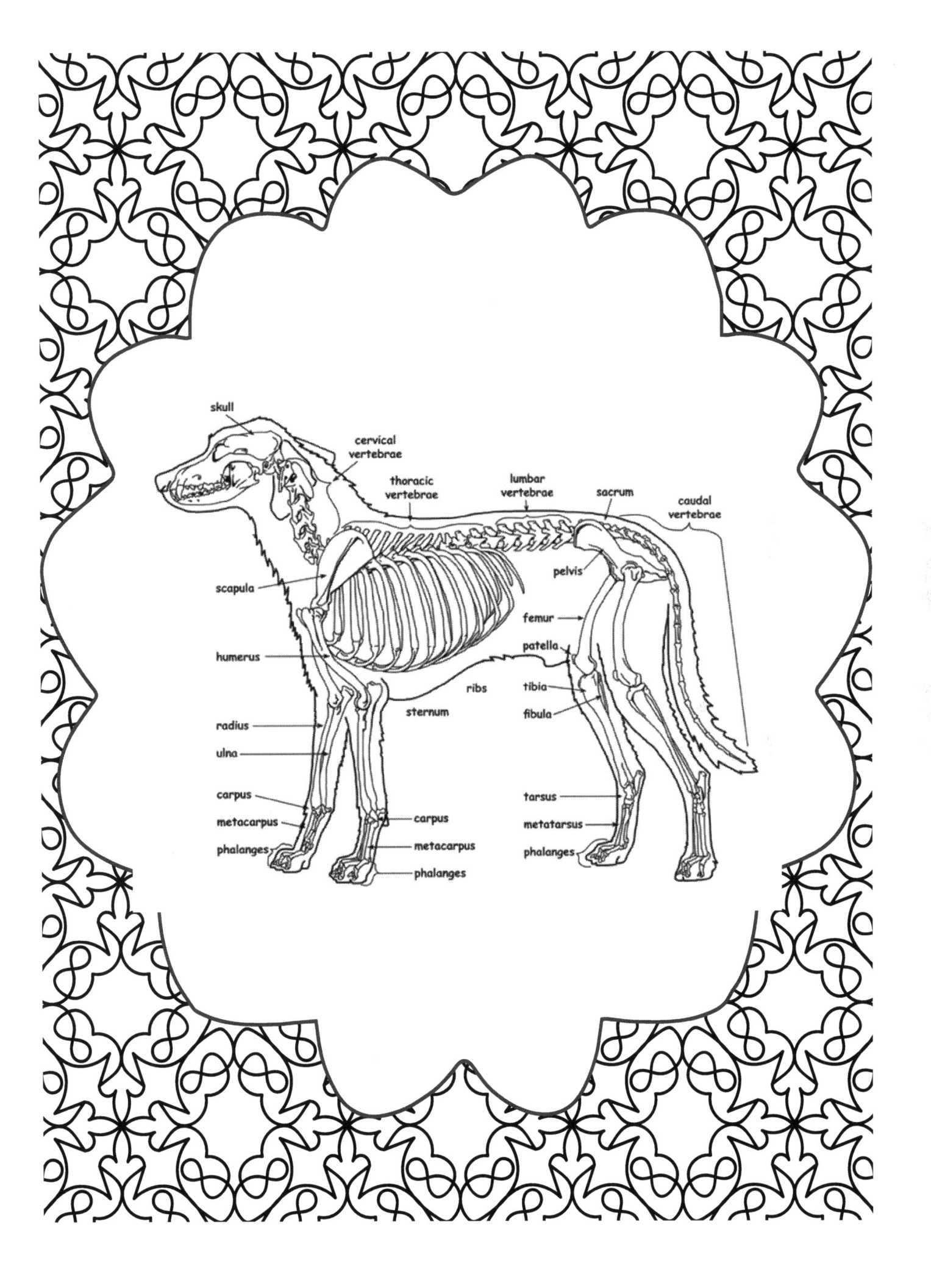

Respiratory System of the Dog

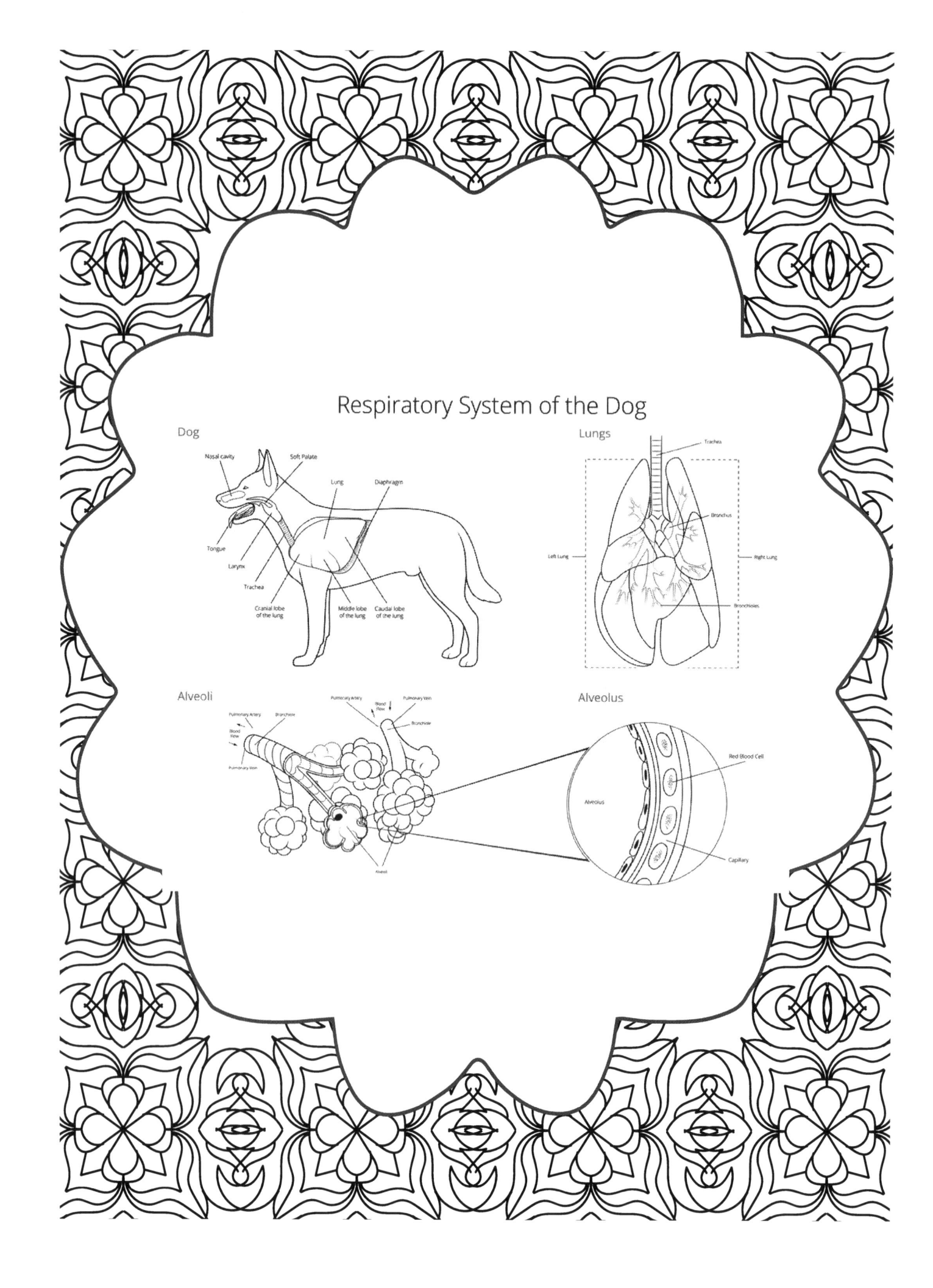

Dog
- Nasal cavity
- Soft Palate
- Lung
- Diaphragm
- Tongue
- Larynx
- Trachea
- Cranial lobe of the lung
- Middle lobe of the lung
- Caudal lobe of the lung

Lungs
- Trachea
- Bronchus
- Left Lung
- Right Lung
- Bronchioles

Alveoli
- Pulmonary Artery
- Bronchiole
- Pulmonary Artery
- Blood Flow
- Pulmonary Vein
- Bronchiole
- Blood Flow
- Pulmonary Vein
- Alveoli

Alveolus
- Red Blood Cell
- Alveolus
- Capillary

ANATOMY OF A PUG

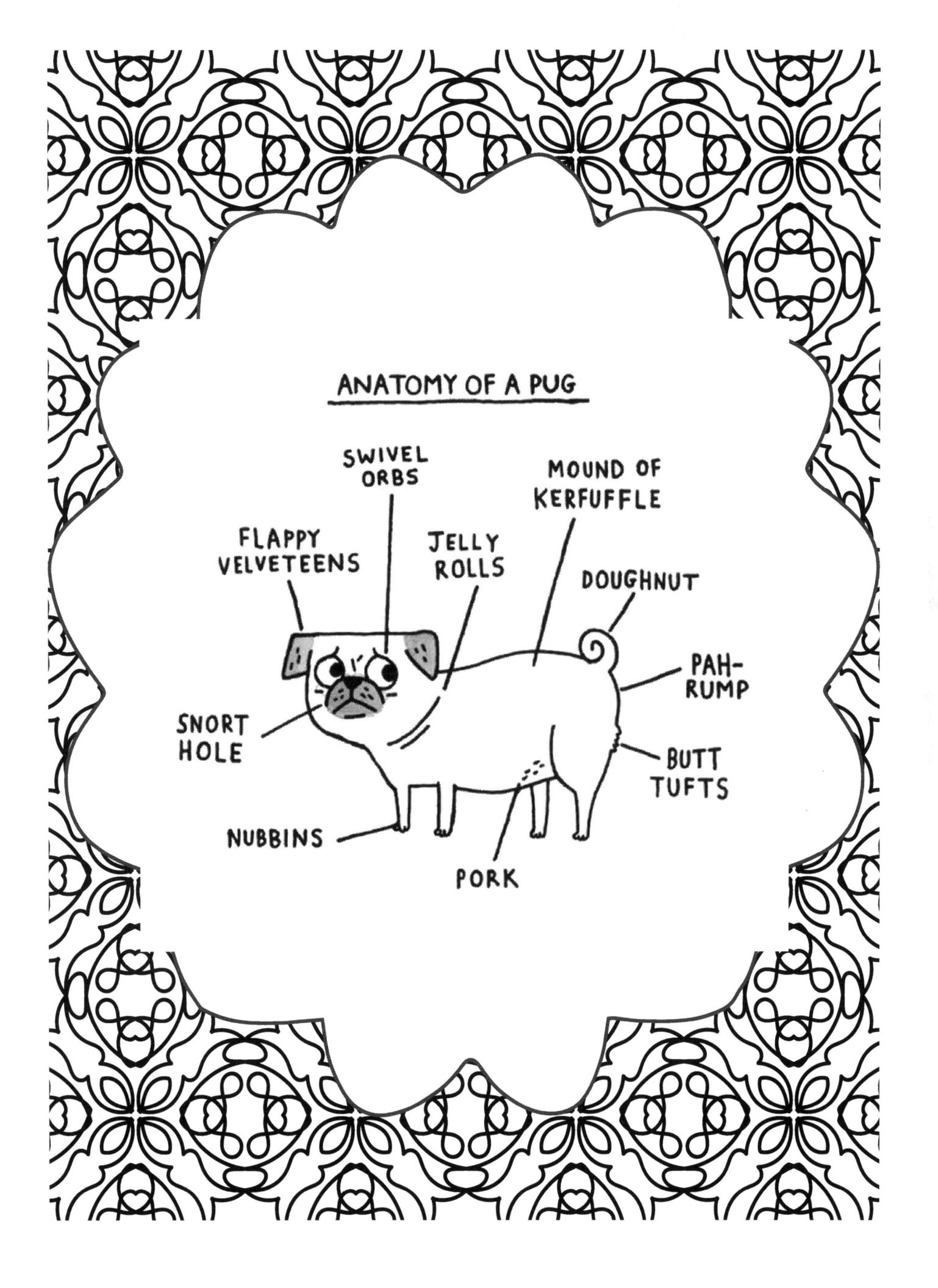

- FLAPPY VELVETEENS
- SWIVEL ORBS
- JELLY ROLLS
- MOUND OF KERFUFFLE
- DOUGHNUT
- PAH-RUMP
- SNORT HOLE
- BUTT TUFTS
- NUBBINS
- PORK

Lungs of the dog

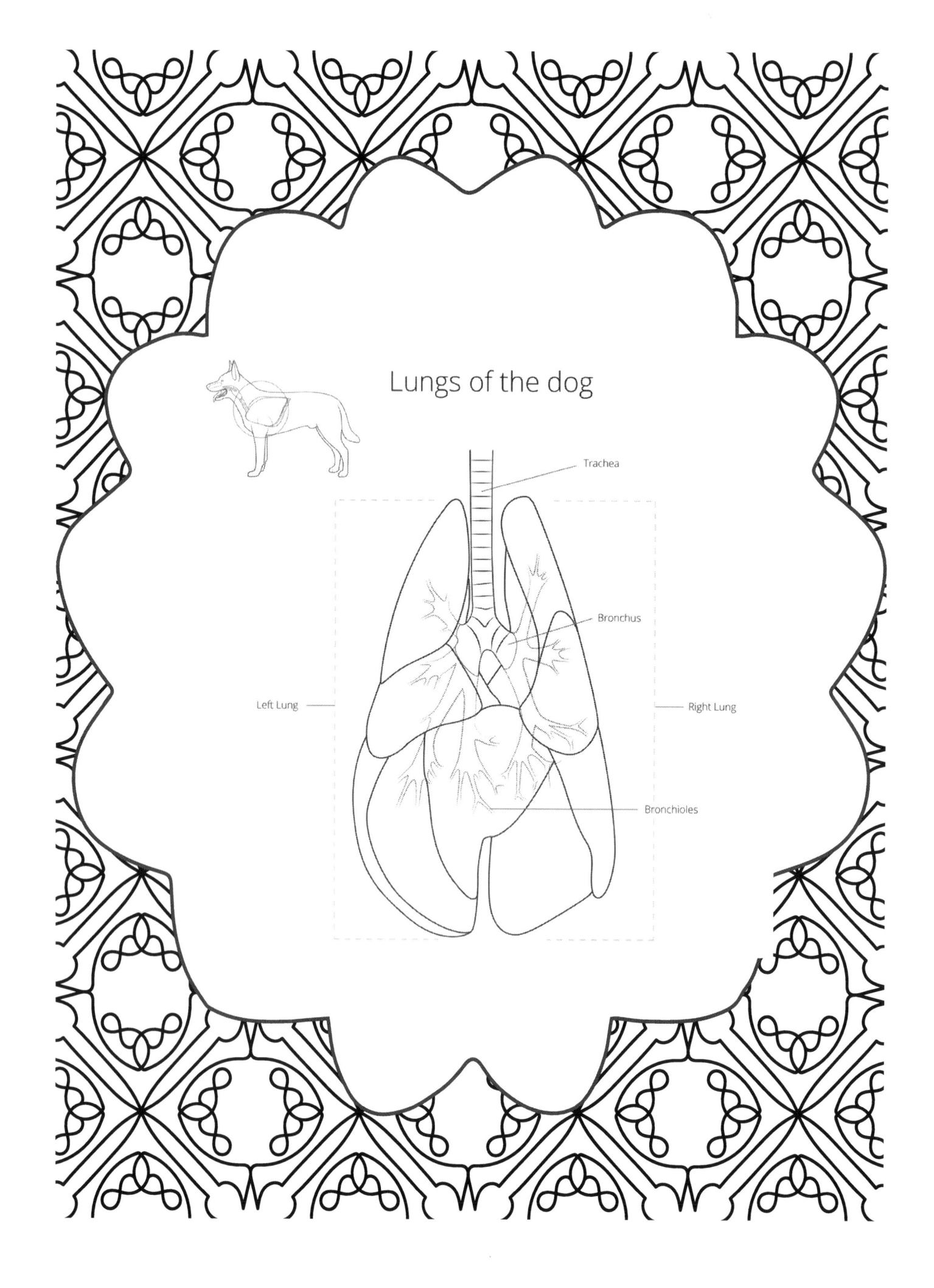

- Trachea
- Bronchus
- Left Lung
- Right Lung
- Bronchioles

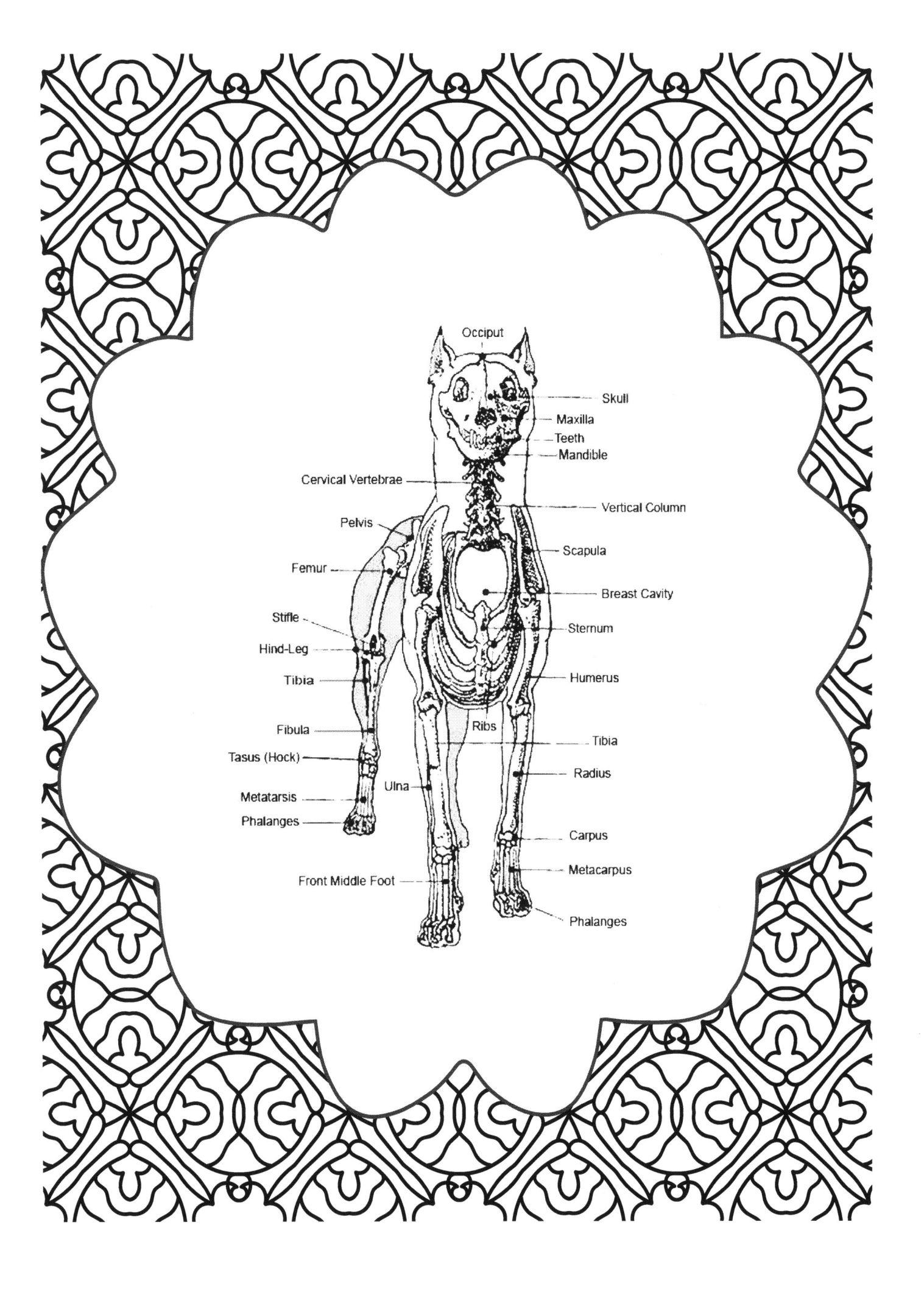

- Occiput
- Skull
- Maxilla
- Teeth
- Mandible
- Cervical Vertebrae
- Vertical Column
- Pelvis
- Scapula
- Femur
- Breast Cavity
- Stifle
- Sternum
- Hind-Leg
- Tibia
- Humerus
- Fibula
- Ribs
- Tibia
- Tasus (Hock)
- Radius
- Metatarsis
- Ulna
- Phalanges
- Carpus
- Metacarpus
- Front Middle Foot
- Phalanges

Bones of the Dog

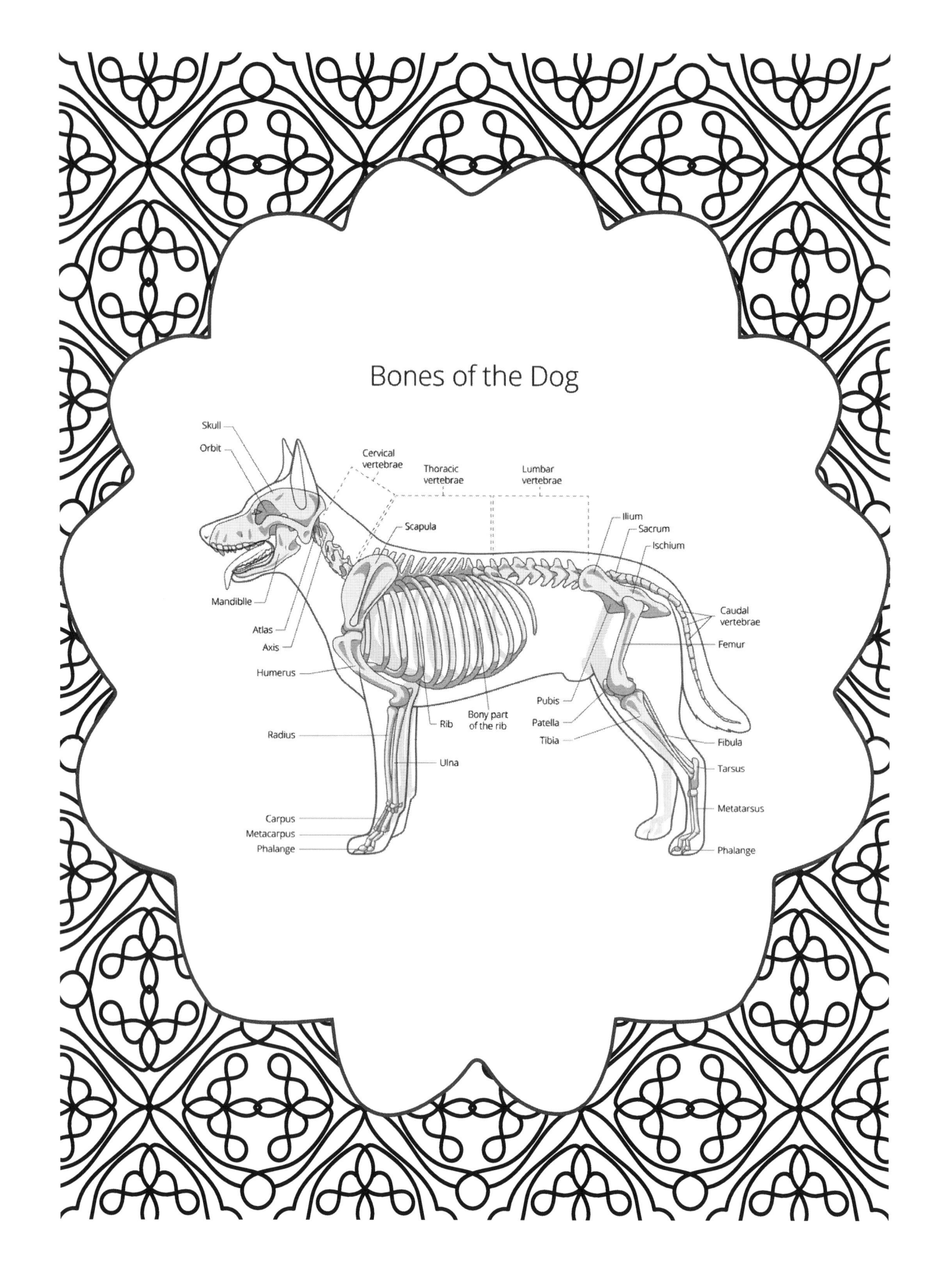

- Skull
- Orbit
- Cervical vertebrae
- Thoracic vertebrae
- Lumbar vertebrae
- Ilium
- Sacrum
- Scapula
- Ischium
- Mandible
- Caudal vertebrae
- Atlas
- Axis
- Femur
- Humerus
- Pubis
- Rib
- Patella
- Bony part of the rib
- Radius
- Tibia
- Fibula
- Ulna
- Tarsus
- Carpus
- Metatarsus
- Metacarpus
- Phalange
- Phalange

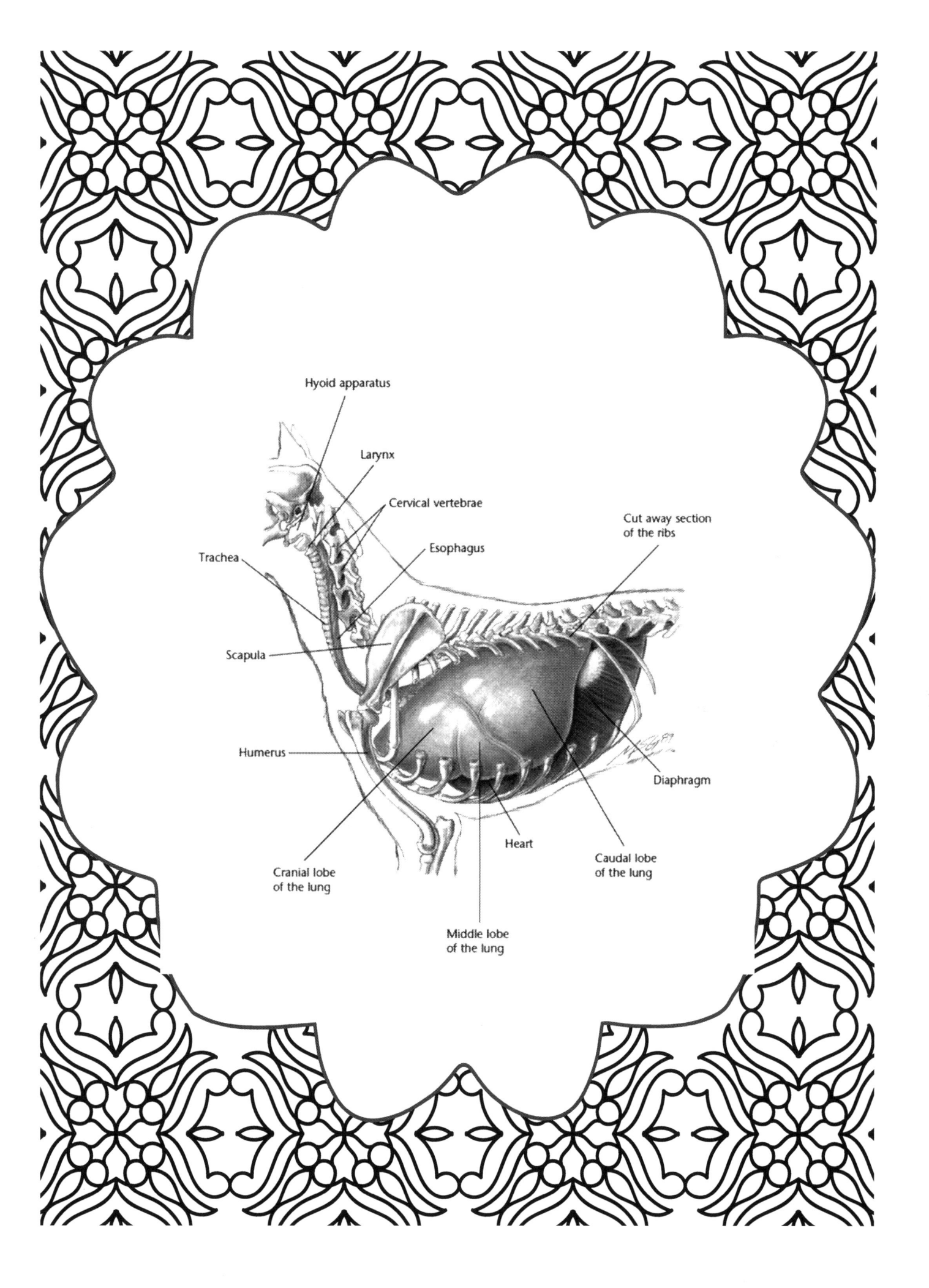

- Hyoid apparatus
- Larynx
- Cervical vertebrae
- Esophagus
- Cut away section of the ribs
- Trachea
- Scapula
- Humerus
- Diaphragm
- Cranial lobe of the lung
- Heart
- Caudal lobe of the lung
- Middle lobe of the lung

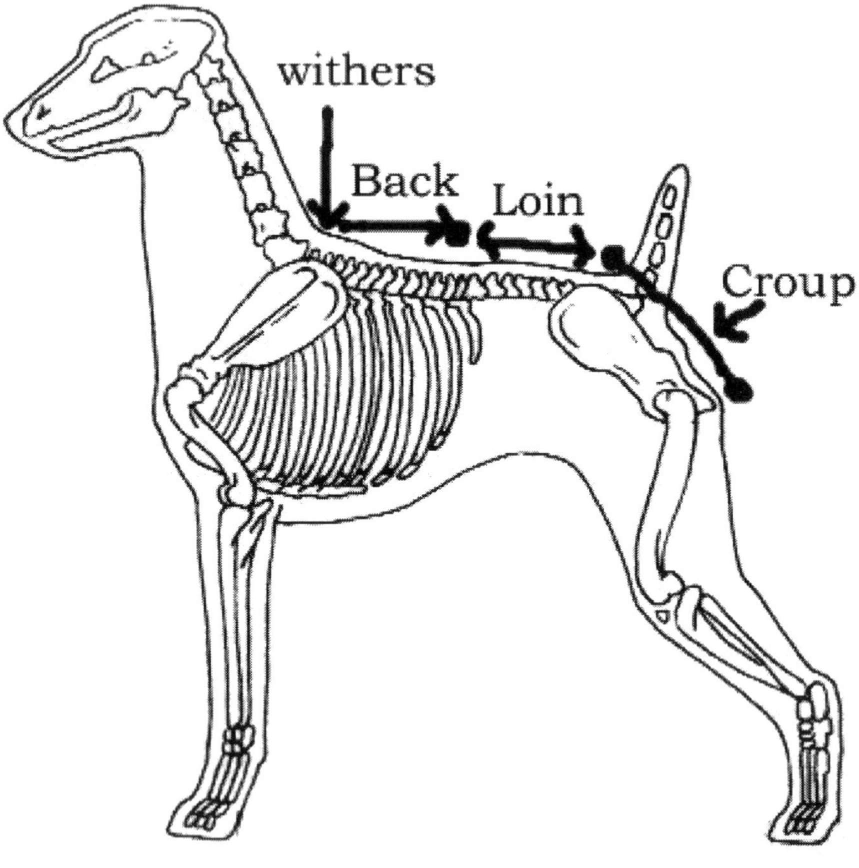
withers
Back
Loin
Croup

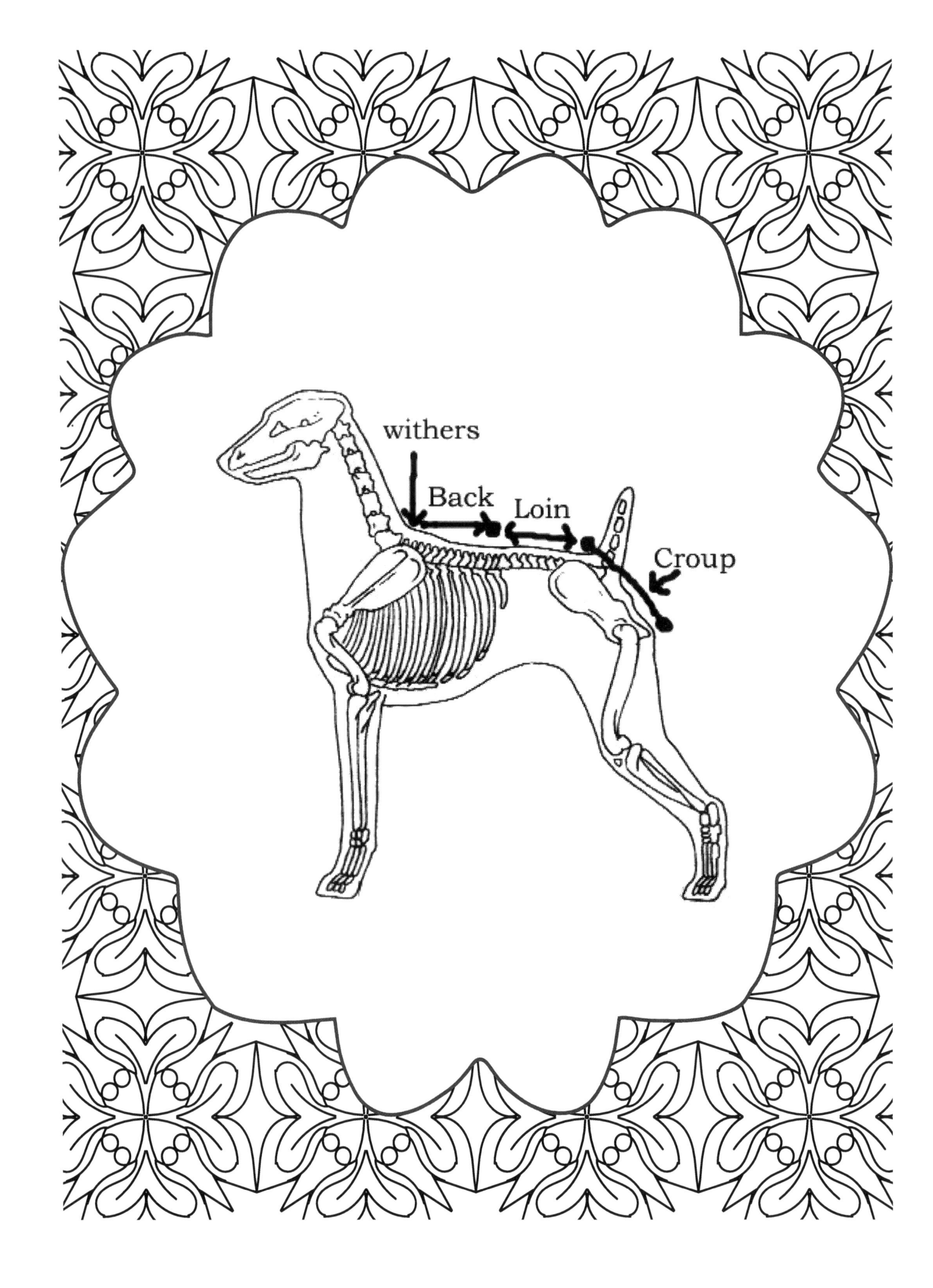

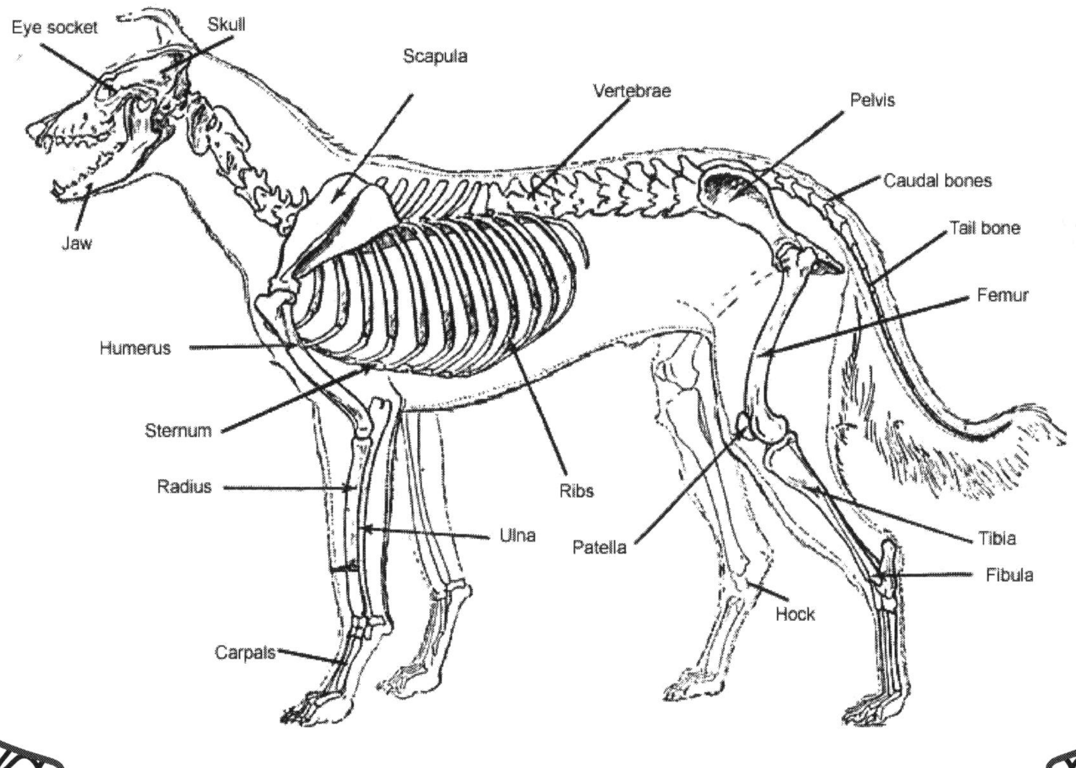
Eye socket
Skull
Scapula
Vertebrae
Pelvis
Caudal bones
Jaw
Tail bone
Femur
Humerus
Sternum
Radius
Ribs
Ulna
Patella
Tibia
Fibula
Hock
Carpals

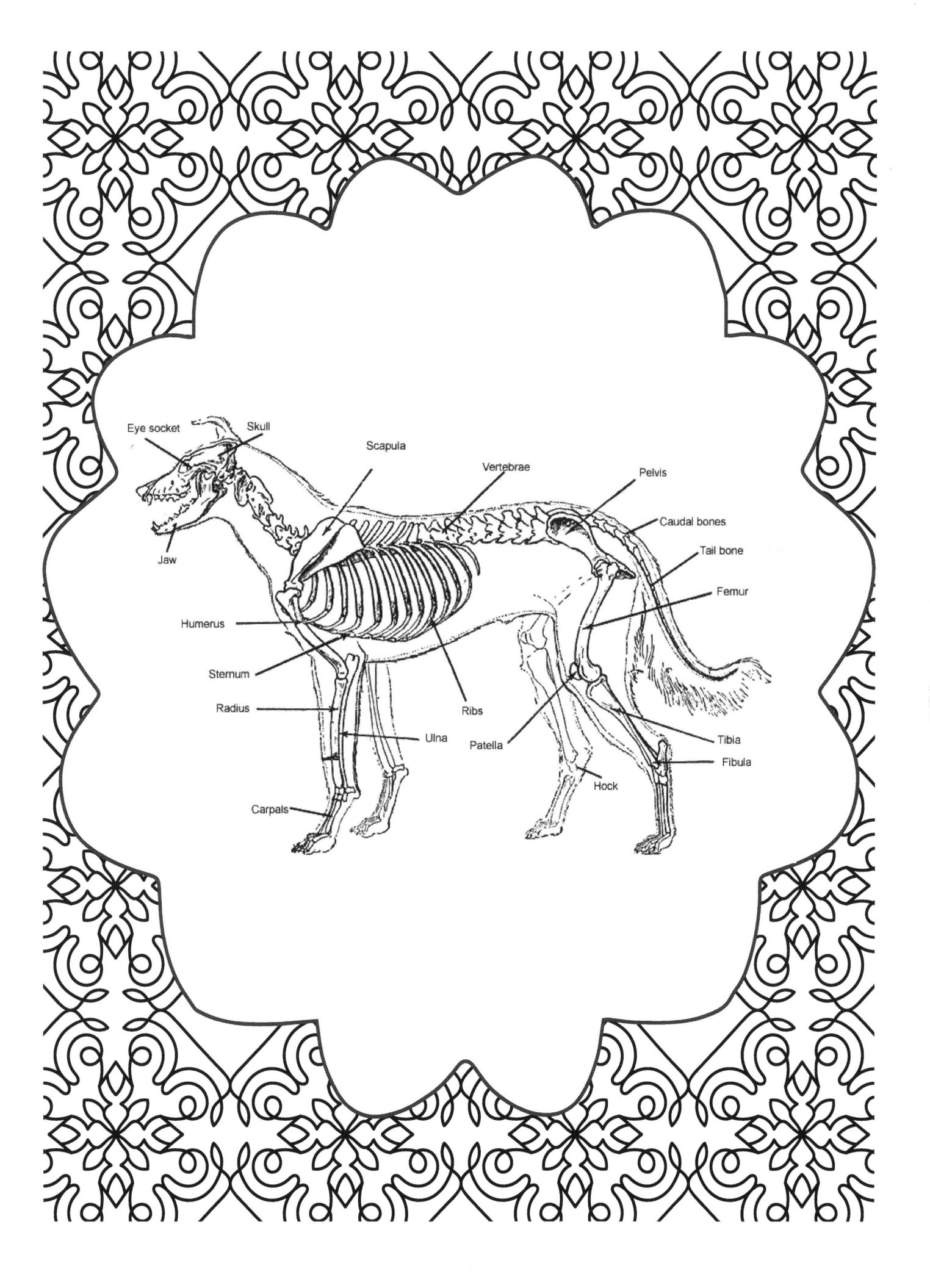

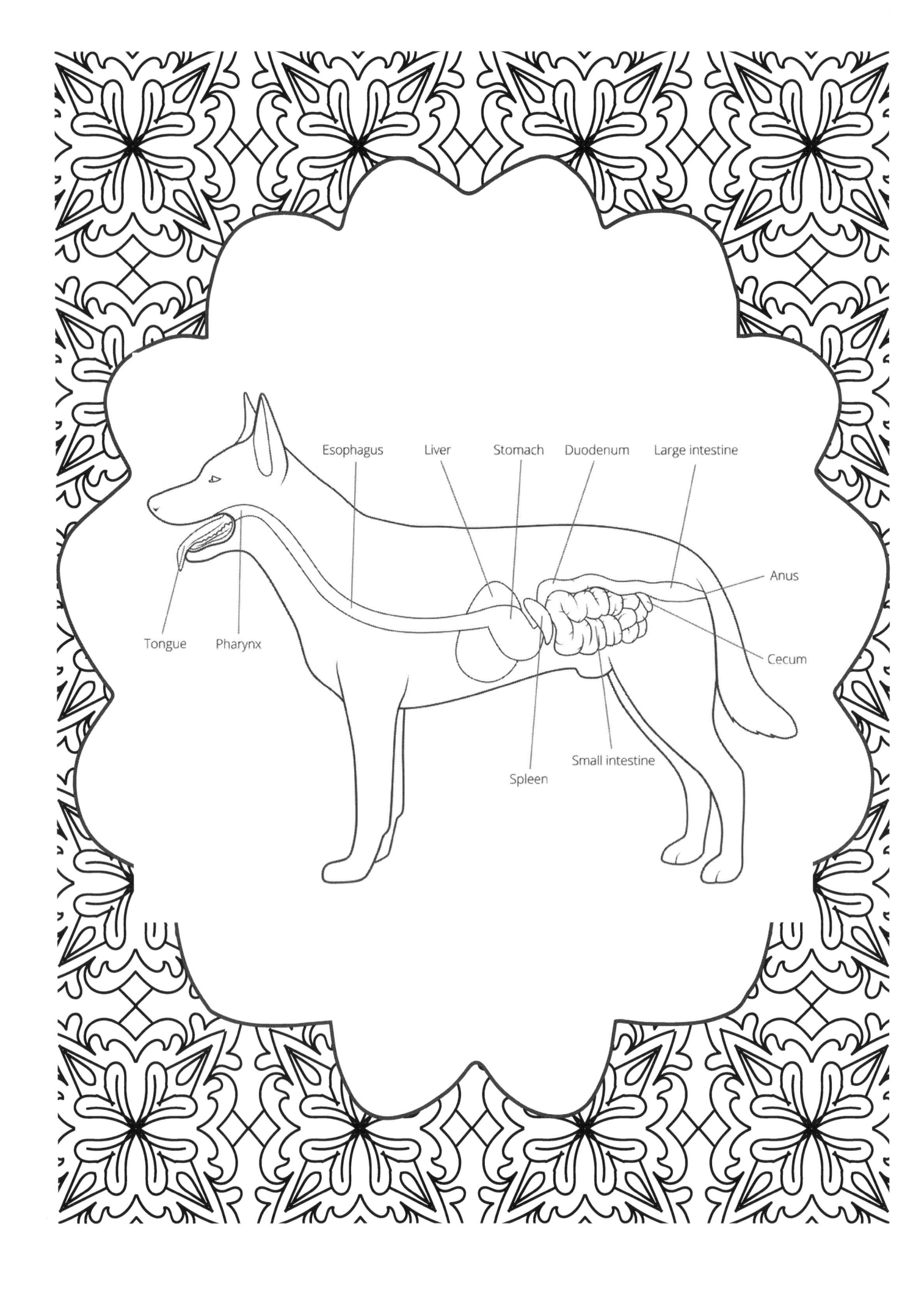

Esophagus · Liver · Stomach · Duodenum · Large intestine

Anus

Cecum

Tongue · Pharynx

Spleen · Small intestine

Made in United States
Orlando, FL
08 February 2023